DR. EARL MINDELL'S

PROBIOTIC

BIBLE

Learn How Healthy Bacteria Can Help Your Body
Absorb Nutrients, Enhance Your Immune System,
and Prevent *and* Treat Disease

Dr. Earl Mindell

TURNER PUBLISHING COMPANY

Turner Publishing Company

Nashville, Tennessee

www.turnerpublishing.com

The information contained in this book is based upon the research and personal and professional experiences of the author. It is not intended as a substitute for consulting with your physician or other healthcare provider. Any attempt to diagnose and treat an illness should be done under the direction of a healthcare professional.

The publisher does not advocate the use of any particular healthcare protocol but believes the information in this book should be available to the public. The publisher and author are not responsible for any adverse effects or consequences resulting from the use of the suggestions, preparations, or procedures discussed in this book. Should the reader have any questions concerning the appropriateness of any procedures or preparations mentioned, the author and the publisher strongly suggest consulting a professional healthcare advisor.

Cover Design: Marc Whitaker
Typesetter: Tim Holtz

Library of Congress Cataloging-in-Publication Data Available Upon Request

Paperback: 9781684423552

Hardcover: 9781684423569

Ebook: 9781684423569

Printed in the United States of America

10 9 8 7 6 5 4 3 2 1

CONTENTS

ACKNOWLEDGMENTS

The author is indebted to Dr. S. K. Dash, the internationally known probiotic pioneer who has made significant contributions to this book.

Dr. Dash is the founder and president of UAS Laboratories, the leading probiotic company since 1979. Dr. Dash has set quality control standards for probiotics (CFU/gm), which are now used worldwide. He is the first to commercialize superstrain DDS-1 *L. acidophilus*, which is acid resistant and bile resistant. He has introduced nitrogen packaging that enables stability of probiotics. Dr. Dash is the first to introduce non-dairy probiotics and fortification of prebiotics (fructooligosaccharides) with probiotics. Dr. Dash's probiotic products, DDS-Probiotics, have been top sellers in the United States and Canada since 1979. DDS-Probiotics are backed by U.S. Trademark, Patent, and medical research and are listed in *Physicians' Desk Reference*.

Dr. Dash says, "A probiotic supplement can only be effective if it contains the right strain(s), in right number (potency), in right condition (viable), and in right formulation." And it must have generally recognized as safe (GRAS) status by the FDA.

According to Dr. Dash, you have to protect probiotics from heat, moisture, and oxygen. For more information about Dr. Dash and his pioneering work, visit www.uaslabs.com.

INTRODUCTION

Antibiotics were first developed in the 1950s. These drugs rapidly attained "miracle drug" status, and for good reason. They cured diseases that had, until then, caused widespread suffering and death, especially in children and the elderly. Right around that time, another miraculous "substance" became available to the public. This substance has been a part of the workings of the human body since it first walked the earth, and has long been a common ingredient in foods known to be healthful. Until the middle of the twentieth century, however, its exact actions in the body were not understood. This substance is *probiotics*—living bacteria that, when supplemented in pill or powder form, take up residence in the body. Once established, these probiotic bacteria perform a variety of functions, all of which promote the physiological balance required for optimal health.

A Brief History of Probiotics

Friendly bacteria have been used to culture milk and other foods since ancient times. Ancient Middle Easterners are known to have regularly consumed yogurt. History texts reveal that, in the early 1200s, the great armies of warlord Genghis Khan made cultured horse milk a staple of their diets. Kefir, another version of fermented milk, originated centuries ago in the Caucasus Mountains of Russia. The bacterial cultures used to make this food, which was widely celebrated as an elixir of health, were highly valued and passed from generation to generation.

In all likelihood, probiotics were discovered by accident when milk was left to sit and was naturally fermented by bacteria. When people discovered that it had a pleasant taste, they probably began to save cultures from particularly good-tasting batches to make more. In this way, the making of yogurt was refined over the centuries.

Around the end of the nineteenth century, a Nobel laureate scientist named Élie Metchnikoff began to wonder why so many members of certain groups of Russian peasants lived for 100 years or more in good health. As he studied their dietary habits, he found that all of these groups regularly consumed milk fermented with friendly bacteria.

After further study, Metchnikoff theorized that the bacteria used to ferment milk had much to do with the longevity of these people. He postulated that most forms of poor health originate in the colon, the part of the body where these good bacteria colonize in the greatest concentrations. Metchnikoff believed that the process of "autointoxication," in which improperly processed wastes seep back through the colon wall into the circulatory system, caused chronic disease. He wrote a book about his discoveries, aptly titled *The Prolongation of Life*.

As early as the 1950s, scientific research began to pile up support for Metchnikoff's ideas, showing that supplementation with probiotics had many beneficial effects. The simultaneous introduction of antibiotics, however, doomed these friendly bacteria to virtual obscurity for several more decades. No matter how well they were able to boost the body's ability to cope with various health problems, they were far overshadowed by quick-acting, potent antibiotics. Probiotics were unable to compete and soon disappeared from the pharmaceutical market.

Today, the growing problem of antibiotic-resistant bacteria has forced medicine to reconsider its overuse of these drugs. The more humans are exposed to antibiotics, the better the dangerous bacteria get at outwitting them. Scaling back the use of these drugs is the only way to preserve their ability to knock out infections—to take the pathogenic bacteria by surprise. Probiotics, the "good" natural enemy of "bad" bacteria, are beginning to enter the picture again as an alternative to antibiotics therapy.

The use of these bacteria, which naturally take up residence in the human body, is an excellent example of alternative medicine's approach to treating illness. Rather than attempting to target and eradicate organisms that cause disease, steps are taken to remedy the imbalance that hampers the body's defenses and allows disease to take hold.

Probiotics aren't exactly nutrients, and they aren't exactly food. They're living bacteria that exist in a symbiotic relationship with the human body. Read on to discover what these microscopic creatures can do to move you toward better health.

CHAPTER 1

FRIENDLY BACTERIA 101

Bacteria are usually viewed as dangerous, unpleasant, unwanted invaders. They lurk on surfaces, spread through airborne droplets emitted during sneezes or coughs, or hide in improperly cooked or spoiled foods. When swallowed or otherwise brought into the body, these bacteria—we are taught to believe—multiply and cause disease. If we can stay away from bacteria, we reason, we can stay free of the illnesses they cause. As soon as a physician suspects a bacterial infection, he or she prescribes antibiotics to get rid of it. Antibacterial soaps, lotions, and cleaning supplies help us in our quest to banish bacteria from our homes and our bodies.

Not all bacteria are bad, however. In fact, there are more than 400 strains of bacteria that are good for your health. These bacteria actually help to resist the growth of pathogens, disease-causing agents. These beneficial bacteria are most commonly known as probiotics. We provide shelter and food to these friendly bugs; they don't live rent-free, however. Our bodies need their services as much as they need ours.

Probiotic bacteria, also known as *intestinal flora, microflora,* and *gut flora,* have been added to milk, soy, and cabbage for centuries. Fermentation with

Antibiotic

Literally, "against life." Refers to drugs administered for the purpose of killing off bacteria that cause symptoms of illness.

Probiotic

Anything that supports life, including food, oxygen, and water. Most commonly refers to more than 400 strains of friendly microorganisms, many of which naturally reside in the body.

Fermentation

The breakdown of complex molecules in organic compounds, caused by the influence of a substance known as a ferment; in the case of yogurt, by friendly microorganisms.

probiotics enhances both shelf life and digestibility of these foods, yielding such delicacies as yogurt, kefir, sour cream, cottage cheese, miso, tempeh, sauerkraut, and kimchee. Modern studies have documented the value of some of these traditional foods for the prevention and treatment of various health problems.

Trillions of Tiny Tenants

The body of a healthy human being provides room and board to a thriving population of more than 400 species of microflora, most of which live in the intestinal tract. In the esophagus and intestines, there are between 1,000 and 1,000,000 bacteria per gram of contents. The large intestine, or colon, provides a cozy home for 100 million to 100 billion probiotic bacteria. All told, these bacteria number about ten times the amount of cells that compose the human body within which they reside—which means that humans are actually 10 percent mammalian cells and 90 percent bacterial cells! These bacteria comprise about 3.5 pounds of the average adult human's body weight.

Babies begin to form this "internal ecosystem" soon after birth. As a baby passes through its mother's birth canal, it receives a dose of the bacteria that populate its mother's vagina. Those bacteria immediately begin to colonize the baby's digestive tract. This could explain why babies born by Cesarean section tend to have more gastrointestinal and other health problems than babies born vaginally. Breast milk contains living probiotics; at this writing, most formulas don't contain these bacteria. This is likely to be one of the reasons why formula is a far inferior food for infants than breast milk, and why it tends to cause colic and other kinds of gastrointestinal upset. For babies who can't be breastfed, supplementation with probiotics has been found to help establish better intestinal health. If you would like to try this with your own child, do so with the guidance of your pediatrician.

What Probiotics Do: An Overview

Probiotics have been found to aid in the prevention or treatment of bacterial infections and viral and fungal infections. They support digestive health in several ways. Growing scientific evidence supports their value in the prevention of certain types of cancer. Maintaining the proper balance of probiotic bacteria has a cleansing effect on the body, which in turn helps prevent diseases that can spring from toxic overload, including autoimmune disease, allergy, and cancer. Efforts to make microflora feel at home in your body will improve your health in many other ways, as well. (Each of these positive effects of probiotics will be addressed in more detail in the chapters to follow.)

- *Probiotics enhance nutrient absorption.* This is one of the most important roles of probiotic bacteria. Without them, the processes that digest, absorb, and detoxify the foods we eat could not proceed smoothly. This is why antibiotics often cause digestive upset; they kill off good bacteria along with bad.

  Amino acids, calcium, zinc, manganese, iron, copper, and phosphorus are all rendered more bioavailable in foods fermented with bacterial cultures. People with lactose intolerance can usually tolerate milk products better when they've been fermented, because the bacteria break down lactose before the food is consumed.

  Many strains of probiotics produce enzymes within the gastrointestinal (GI tract. These enzymes help to break down the foods we eat more completely. The nutrients from these foods can then be better absorbed, and bloating and gas are reduced.

  Intestinal infections can cause diarrhea, constipation, bloating, heartburn, gas, and indigestion. Competition from beneficial bacteria decreases the likelihood that these infections will take hold.

  Many of the most abundant probiotics have an acidifying effect on the gastrointestinal tract. When intestinal pH is close to neutral, as it tends to be in those whose probiotic populations are lacking, the growth of yeasts and unfriendly bacteria is encouraged; increased acidity has the opposite effect. By decreasing pH, microflora improve the passage of nutrients through the intestinal walls and into the bloodstream.

- *Probiotics manufacture nutrients.* Intestinal flora makes an important contribution to optimal nutrition by producing B-complex vitamins, including biotin, thiamine (B_1), riboflavin (B_2), pantothenic acid (B_5), and pyridoxine (B_6). It also produces short-chain fatty acids, antioxidants, amino acids, and vitamin K, which is gaining increasing recognition for its role in bone-building and heart health.

Antibodies

Immune substances specially designed to identify and attack specific pathogens.

- *Probiotics boost immune function.* Probiotics stimulate antibody production and increase the activity of white blood cells, the immune cells that target, consume, and engulf pathogens. They also positively modify the production of *cytokines,* substances immune cells use to communicate with one another.

- *Probiotics slow cancer growth.* Animal studies have shown that pro-biotics can help suppress the growth of cancerous tumors induced by toxic chemicals. Probiotics also inhibit the action of substances that transform healthy cells into cancerous ones, and reduce levels of enzymes that transform precarcinogens into carcinogens. Friendly bacteria seem to be especially good at protecting against colon cancer.

- *Probiotics fight infection.* Gut flora produces chemicals that kill off less friendly "bad" bacteria. Probiotics also suppress the growth of bacteria, yeasts, and viruses by acidifying the digestive tract ("bad" bacteria need a more neutral pH to thrive) and by competing with them for space and resources. They may also work to eliminate pathogenic bacteria by inhibiting their attachment to tissues or by inhibiting "bad" bacteria from secreting toxins.

pH

A measurement of acidity or alkalinity of a solution. A substance with a pH below 7 is an acid; a pH above 7 is a base; a pH of 7 is neutral.

Acid: A substance with a pH below 7.

Base: A substance with a pH above 7.

Neutral: A substance with a pH of 7.

- *Probiotics help prevent food allergies.* Research has shown that probiotics are useful for food sensitivities. They are a crucial part of what's known as the *gut defense barrier*—combined elements of the immune system that cooperate to prevent the absorption of any substance that shouldn't move into the bloodstream. Probiotics are believed to reduce intestinal inflammation, which leads to the formation of the tiny "holes" in the intestinal wall that can allow large food particles into the circulation. The immune system reacts to rid the body of these foreign particles, and this state of immune reactivity can exaggerate allergic reactions to foods and environmental allergens.

- *Probiotics fight yeast overgrowth.* Yeasts—in particular, one strain of yeast known as *Candida albicans*—are natural residents of the digestive tract and mucous membranes throughout the body. When microflora is abundant and the immune system is functioning well, these yeasts are kept in check. They can quickly become overgrown when probiotic populations fall due to antibiotic or synthetic hormone use, or to an overabundance of refined carbohydrates in the diet.

  Yeast infections can affect the vagina, the urinary tract, the mouth and throat, the breasts of lactating women, skin, toenails, and sinuses, or can spread throughout the body. Compromised immunity—an issue for people who are undergoing cancer treatments or who have a disease that hampers immune function—sets the stage for severe systemic yeast overgrowth. In people who are often afflicted by localized yeast infections, a systemic infection is probably at the root of their problem.

- *Probiotics prevent and treat diarrhea and constipation.* Much of the research on probiotics has focused on their use as a therapy for diarrheal diseases, especially in children. High colon pH has been linked with constipation, and lowering pH (making it more acidic) has been found to relieve this condition.

- *Probiotics prevent and treat halitosis.* Chronic bad breath is usually the result of an imbalance of good and bad bacteria in the upper gastrointestinal tract.

- *Probiotics prevent and treat ulcers and stomach cancer.* Ulcers are now known to be caused by the *H. pylori* bacteria, which have also been linked to increases in stomach cancer risk. When good bacteria are present in sufficient numbers, they protect the stomach lining against *H. pylori*.

- *Probiotics prevent and treat inflammatory bowel disease (IBD).* Research supports the use of supplemental probiotics for Crohn's disease, ulcerative colitis, and irritable bowel syndrome. Often, these disorders are directly related to an imbalanced internal ecosystem, and making adjustments to boost probiotic populations goes a long way toward restoring balance in the colon.

Why Probiotic Levels Fall

Once upon a time, humankind managed to maintain adequate probiotic counts without any kind of supplement. Although foods fermented with friendly flora have been eaten around the world throughout history, many civilizations managed without those foods. What's different today? Why do so many people need to consider the use of a supplemental source of probiotics?

1. Many children are born by C-section and are fed formula, both of which hamper the initial development of healthy probiotic populations.

2. Modern humans consume millions of times fewer *Lactobacilli* and other friendly flora than our Paleolithic ancestors did.

3. Diets rich in refined carbohydrates and sugars—all too common in children and adults—enhance the growth of "bad" bacteria and yeasts, to the detriment of the friendly bacteria. Diets that are heavy on the meat and light on the vegetables and fruits alter the activity of friendly bacteria. Plant foods contain *prebiotics*, the favorite foods of probiotics; in fact, the best probiotic supplements contain prebiotics. (More on this in Chapter 9.)

4. Chlorinated water has damaging effects on friendly bacteria.

5. Exposure to antibiotic drugs depletes probiotics throughout the body. Antibiotic drugs don't only kill off the bad guys. They do a clean sweep of the body's good bacteria, as well.

6. The frequent use of antacids and other acid- reducing drugs lower the acidity of the gastrointestinal (GI) tract, which creates an inhospitable environment for friendly bacteria.

7. Synthetic estrogens taken in the form of birth control pills or hormone replacement also decrease microflora populations. This is why the use of antibiotic drugs can cancel out the effects of birth control pills and cause breakthrough bleeding in premenopausal women.

8. Oral steroid drugs such as Prednisone and inhaled steroid drugs for asthma decrease probiotic counts.

9. Friendly bacteria are sensitive to their host's stress levels. Stress alters the balance of important hormones, and this shift can cause probiotic populations to dwindle.

Read on to discover exactly how lack of microflora can harm your health, and how restoring optimal probiotic balance can relieve many common health problems.

CHAPTER 2

PROBIOTICS AND UPPER DIGESTIVE TRACT HEALTH

Although probiotics have multiple roles throughout the body, their most important duties involve the health of the gastrointestinal (GI) tract. If your digestive system isn't functioning well, the fallout affects every part of your body. The health of every cell that makes up who you are is dependent upon the ability of your mouth, esophagus, stomach, small intestines, and large intestines to extract the nutrients from the foods you eat and get rid of what's indigestible or toxic. Chronically disrupted digestion not only can cause outright and uncomfortable symptoms—including bad breath, indigestion, gas, bloating, flatulence, constipation, and diarrhea—it can have more subtle effects caused by the body's inability to move nutrients out of the GI tract to the parts of the body where they're needed for cellular operations.

In this chapter and the following one, you will learn about the roles of friendly microorganisms all along the digestive tract. When you see how much responsibility these microscopic bugs take on, you'll want to do all you can to support them and boost their populations.

A Party in Your Mouth

Breath-freshening gum, candy, and mouthwash are all big business in the Western world. These products temporarily mask bad breath, and some kill off bacteria that create unpleasant odors. What they don't do is improve the ecosystem within the mouth—an ecosystem that, when properly maintained, can keep breath odor-free without any hint of over-powering "minty freshness."

Each milliliter of saliva is populated by anywhere from 10,000 to 1 billion microorganisms. Among the residents of your mouth are friendly streptococci, lactobacilli, veillonella, bacteroides, fusobacteria, staph-ylococci, and cornybacteria. These microorganisms produce acids and antibacterial substances that prevent colonization by unfriendly yeasts and bacteria—critters that manufacture toxins that can be at the root of chronic cases of bad breath (halitosis).

When friendly flora populations fall, putrefying bacteria can overpop-ulate the upper GI tract. As you might guess from the term "putrefying," this can alter the odor of a person's breath for the worse. According to probiotics expert Dr. S. K. Dash, unfriendly bacterial overpopulation can also contribute to canker sores and belching—two more problems that tend to hamper one's social life. Bringing mouth and throat microorgan-isms back into balance can remedy all of these issues.

If your breath seems unpleasant despite constant use of breath-fresh-ening gum, candy, or mouthwash, try rinsing your mouth and gargling with probiotic solution. Or, you can pour the contents of a probiotic cap-sule or tablet in your mouth and hold it there for as long as you can before swallowing. These tactics will help to give good bacteria the edge in your mouth.

Don't Suppress Stomach Acid to Cure Ulcers

The stomach is a dangerous place for all types of bacteria, friendly and unfriendly alike. Within this organ, the pH naturally falls between 1 and 3, and most pathogens are destroyed by this powerful acidity. In a healthy GI tract, only acid-resistant bacteria, such as the beneficial *Lacto-bacilli* and *Bifidobacterium,* consistently survive the journey through the stomach. However, all probiotic bacteria are not acid and bile resistant.

Antacids and acid-reducing drugs are big business these days. Main-stream medicine's tack for treating reflux involves buffering acid with antacids such as Tums or suppressing acid production with drugs such as Tagamet (ranitidine) or Zantac (cimetidine). In most instances, however, gastroesophageal reflux disease (GERD) and related issues result not from too much acid, but from *too little.* Medical research has shown that low acid production is a very common problem, and is thought in some research circles to affect half

GERD

A condition in which acid from the stomach leaks up into the esophagus.

the people over the age of sixty. Other research suggests that asthma, acne rosacea, and rheumatoid arthritis may be related to low stomach acidity.

Treating heartburn and acid reflux with acid-reducing therapies might relieve immediate discomfort, but over time it's making the problem worse by making the stomach a more hospitable place for the growth of unfriendly bacteria. Low acid secretion also hampers the absorption of important vitamins and minerals, including folate, B_6, B_{12}, iron, and calcium.

It's true that eating heavy, fatty meals can cause stomach acid *oversecretion*, but cutting down on troublesome foods can solve this problem far more safely than acid-reducing drugs can.

Ulcers were once thought to be caused by spicy foods and stress, and they were treated with bland diet and acid-reducing drugs. Recent research breakthroughs have shown that most ulcers are caused by a more complex group of factors, including an acid-resistant bacteria called *Helicobacter pylori* (*H. pylori*). It is believed that more than 50 percent of people harbor *H. pylori*, and that in a balanced gastrointestinal ecosystem it does no harm. When

Gastric Ulcer

Erosions in the mucous lining of the stomach that allow powerful acids to come into contact with and injure unprotected tissues beneath that lining.

its populations grow more than they should, this bug contributes to the formation of ulcers, and has been linked with stomach cancer, chronic stomach inflammation (gastritis), heart disease, and autoimmune disease.

Mainstream medicine uses three or four antibiotics simultaneously to treat *H. pylori* infection. Evidence shows that those who are infected with *H. pylori* are also more likely to have an overgrowth of the yeast *Candida albicans*, the one that most often causes yeast infections. *H. pylori* and *C. albicans* appear to have a symbiotic relationship, where the yeast actually helps to protect the ulcer-causing bacteria against antibiotics. During the course of intensive antibiotic treatment—really the only way to eradicate this bug—good bacteria are killed off, leaving the gastrointestinal environment even more vulnerable to overgrowth of pathogens. Chances are good that either a resistant form of *H. pylori* or some other infection will reemerge once the antibiotic therapy is complete.

Probiotics won't cure ulcers, but some probiotic bacteria (*L. acidophilus, L. casei, L. bulgaricus, B. bifidus, Pediococcus pentosaceus*) have been found to inhibit *H. pylori* growth in laboratory experiments. Using a probiotic supplement regularly throughout treatment for *H. pylori* infection will support recovery by continually re-establishing friendly bacterial populations. It's best to continue to take the probiotics for a week or two after the completion of antibiotic therapy.

Probiotics Improve Digestion

Difficulty digesting the sugars in milk, known as *lactose*, is often behind otherwise unexplained gastrointestinal symptoms, such as gas, bloating, and diarrhea. Probiotics break down lactose in dairy products before they ever pass through your lips. This is why many lactose intolerant people find that they can digest live-culture yogurt and acidophilus milk without problems.

Many strains of probiotics manufacture enzymes within the GI tract. These enzymes aid in the complete breakdown of the foods we eat. When enzymes do the job in the small intestines, the nutrients in those foods are better absorbed, and the likelihood of undigested food particles passing into the colon to be broken down by microflora—and producing gas, bloating, and flatulence—is less.

Friendly Bacteria Protect Against Leaky Gut

Researchers have found that the foods we eat have strong effects on the function of the small intestine. This organ is a narrow tube, about twenty feet in length, lined with tissues that are specially designed to absorb needed nutrients into the bloodstream. From there, those nutrients are distributed to wherever they are needed in the body. Along the small intestine's inner surface, both physical and immunological barriers do their best to prevent the passage of any potentially harmful substance into the circulation. Probiotics are an important element of this barrier.

Processed food diets throw these small intestinal barriers out of whack. Diets loaded with fatty meat and dairy, processed flour, and sugar gum up the muscular contractions that move food through the intestines. This increases *transit time*—the amount of time it takes for a meal to be completely digested and wastes excreted. Slowed transit time and impaired intestinal contractions both disrupt the integrity of the intestinal wall by enhancing the growth of bad bacteria and creating pockets of inflammation. On a typical American diet, probiotic bacteria suffer as the natural flow of the nutrients they require is reduced. The upshot: standard dietary fare alters the small intestinal balance of good and bad bacteria for the worse.

This imbalance can lead to the development of openings in the lining of the small intestine—a condition known as *leaky gut.* Large particles that wouldn't normally move into the bloodstream are able to do so, and the immune system targets them as foreign and mounts an attack on them, resulting in a constant state of inflammation that shows up in the multifarious form of food allergy symptoms. At the same time, disrupted intestinal ecology leads to an overproduction of the toxins that are manufactured by bad bacteria. Those toxins can create more "holes" in the gut, and the immune system has to deal with them in the bloodstream, as well. The use of NSAIDs (nonsteroidal anti-inflammatory drugs, such as ibuprofen, aspirin, and the COX-2 inhibitor drugs celecoxib and rofecoxib) may cause or worsen leaky gut; aging, alcoholism, or bacterial infections may also contribute. If you suspect that your gut is leaky, a naturopathically oriented physician can confirm your suspicions with a *lactulose/mannitol* test.

Food Allergy

When a food component—most often, a protein—elicits an immune response.

The most commonly allergenic foods are eggs, milk, peanuts, soy, and wheat. Beef, pork, and veal are allergenic in some people. If you have one or more of the following health problems, food allergies may be at least partially to blame:

- Irritable bowel syndrome
- Colitis
- Constipation
- Diarrhea
- Bladder infections
- Asthma
- Acne
- Skin rashes/unexplained itching
- Low-functioning immune system, resulting in frequent infections
- Depression
- Anxiety
- Mental confusion

- Insomnia

- Joint/low back pain

- Irregular heartbeat (arrhythmia)

- Fatigue

- Headaches/migraines

- Sinusitis

- Hypoglycemia

Good Bacteria Control Yeast Overgrowth

Yeasts are natural inhabitants of the human ecosystem, particularly the intestines and vaginal and urinary tracts. One type of yeast is especially opportunistic when friendly flora populations dwindle: *Candida albicans*, also known as *C. albicans* or candida.

When beneficial flora are more scarce—killed off by poor diet, antibiotics, steroid drugs, or oral contraceptives—candida undergoes a Jekyll-and-Hyde-style transformation, from a benign yeast to an insidious fungus. In scientific terms, this Mr. Hyde is referred to as the yeast's *mycelial fungal* form. When in this form, candida sprouts offshoots called *rhizoids*, which can penetrate the walls of the intestines. Many experts believe that this transformation is responsible for most cases of leaky gut, and for the assault on the immune system that results as foreign particles pass into the bloodstream. Candida in this form can spread throughout the body, causing a systemic yeast infection, or *candidiasis*. The immune system reacts to this shift by mounting an attack against the invasive yeast. Over time, this heightened state of immune reactivity drains the body and can aggravate allergies, autoimmune disease, and other health problems related to an off-kilter immune system.

Yeast infections can show up in the vagina, mouth, throat, or urinary tract, or on the skin and nails. Nursing mothers often develop yeast infections in their nipples, and nursing infants are prone to oral thrush. Although these infections seem localized, they are often a sign that a systemic infection needs attention.

Mainstream medicine has long believed that candidiasis only affects seriously immunocompromised people, such as AIDS sufferers or chemotherapy patients. According to experts in the natural health field—including William Crook, M.D., (author of *The Yeast Connection*) and

C. Orian Truss (author of *The Missing Diagnosis*)—candida overgrowth is much more common than previously thought, largely due to widespread overuse of antibiotics and oral contraceptives.

Convincing scientific evidence has linked candidiasis with a long list of common health complaints that have defied conventional explanations, including depression, anxiety, irritability, chronic heartburn or indigestion, bloating, reflux disease, constipation, difficulty concentrating, flatulence, fatigue, allergies to foods or environmental factors, migraines, cystitis, acne, and chronic menstrual complaints. If you tend to have repeated bouts of vaginal yeast infection, cystitis, urinary tract infection, eczema, psoriasis, oral thrush, or toenail fungus, a few steps to control systemic candida are probably necessary.

First, change your diet. Eliminate all sugars and refined carbohydrates (white bread, cake, cookies, white pasta). Avoid fruits and juices, which are high in natural sugars. Fermented foods, including beer, wine, cheese, vinegar, sour cream, buttermilk, tofu, soy sauce, miso, and cider, should be avoided. Mushrooms should also be cut from the anti-yeast diet.

Traditionally, severe candidiasis has been treated with antifungal medications such as Nystatin. While drugs will wipe out the yeast infection, it's likely to return if diet and lifestyle changes conducive to optimal probiotic populations aren't made. The most current therapies for candida overgrowth include *reinoculation*—supplying the body with enough supplemental proven probiotics to bring the internal ecosystem back into balance—and high doses (300 mg/day) of the B vitamin biotin. *Caprylic acid* is a naturally occurring fatty acid that is lethal to candida and can be bought over the counter. Garlic and the herb Pau d'arco are also helpful when it comes to bringing candida back under control.

You can use probiotics to treat both systemic and local invasion of candida. Take higher doses of proven probiotic supplements daily to repopulate your GI tract with these candida-busting microorganisms. For vaginal yeast infections, try a plain yogurt douche or a moistened tampon sprinkled with active probiotic culture and left in place overnight. Yogurt or probiotic solution (probiotic powder mixed with water to make a thin paste) can be applied to the vaginal area to soothe irritated tissues. Repeated sinus infections may be related to local candida overgrowth; to remedy this, try sniffing a watery solution of probiotics into each nostril. For oral thrush in children or adults—this is a common side effect of inhaled steroid drugs for asthma or allergies—pour the contents of a probiotic capsule or tablet into the mouth and hold it there for as long as possible before swallowing. For nursing infants, a dusting of probiotic powder (use one designed for babies) on mom's nipple before a nursing session should help. Or, try a probiotic solution made with breast milk or water, to be swabbed into the inside of baby's mouth. Applying probiotic solution to the nipples will also help to clear up yeast-related breast infections.

Toenail fungus may respond well to overall balancing of the internal ecosystem. If you have this problem, you can try applying probiotic solution directly to the affected areas. Topical garlic and tea tree oil have also been recommended for treatment of toenail fungus.

The health of the small intestines play a crucial role in the overall health of the body. A "leaky" intestinal tract can also throw a wrench in the works by causing chronic inflammation throughout the body or specific inflammatory problems such as allergies, asthma, and autoimmune disease. Probiotics help to prevent these problems by maintaining the gut lining and modulating the gut immune system.

CHAPTER 3

COLON HEALTH
AND PROBIOTICS

Near the end of the nineteenth century, many believed that ill health during old age could be traced back to *autointoxication*. Wastes and toxins from the colon were thought to seep into the bloodstream, poisoning the body and setting chronic disease processes in motion. According to this theory, colon cleansing is an integral part of both disease prevention and disease treatment. Modern, technological medicine has rejected these ideas, but natural medicine has maintained that vibrant good health does rely, at least in part, on the condition of the colon (also known as the large intestine). Although this organ and its functions aren't exactly a polite topic of conversation, its importance in the maintenance of optimal health is undeniable.

The colon plays a complex role in the processing of nutrients and hormones. It provides a home for between 100 million and 100 billion friendly microorganisms, including *Bacteroides spp.*, *Fusobacterium spp.*, *Lactobacilli*, and *Bifidobacteria*. Less friendly inhabitants such as *Clostridium* and *Salmonella* are sometimes found in the colon, but when this organ is in its healthy state, they don't survive long.

Probiotic bacteria have a number of tactics for inhibiting the growth of pathogens throughout the GI tract. They produce at least three substances that wipe out bad bacteria: *acidophilin*, a natural antibiotic that kills off dangerous strains of *E. coli, streptococcus,* and *staphylococcus* bacteria; *lactic acid,* which creates an inhospitable acidic environment for pathogens; and *hydrogen peroxide,* a free radical used by the immune system to do battle with unwanted invaders. Probiotics also directly boost immune function, which I'll tell you more about in Chapter 4.

When the balance of good and bad microorganisms in the colon is chronically out of whack—a state of affairs known as *dysbiosis*—unfriendly bacteria can grow unfettered. Overgrowth of pathogenic bacteria and yeasts leads to the production of toxic byproducts that pass through the colon wall and into the circulation.

The Colon's Roles in Digestion

Probiotics in the colon complete the digestive process by breaking down complex molecules that can't be dismantled anywhere else in the GI tract. Electrolytes and water are reabsorbed through the walls of the colon. The cells that line the colon are replaced completely every week, and this process requires a lot of energy; they don't receive nutrients from the bloodstream as most tissues do, however. Vitamins, minerals, and accessory nutrients needed by this organ are all made by the probiotics that live along its walls. Arginine, cysteine, glutamine, B vitamins (thiamine, riboflavin, pantothenic acid, and pyridoxine), antioxidants, and vitamin K are produced by gut bacteria in the colon. Electrolytes and water are also absorbed back through the colon walls.

> **Electrolytes**
>
> Minerals such as magnesium, chloride, potassium, and sodium, needed to conduct the electricity that powers nerve impulses and muscle contraction and release.

The colon is about five feet long and two and a half inches in diameter. Once a meal has passed through the small intestines, most of the nutrients it contained have been absorbed through the intestinal wall. Your body isn't content to let the rest of your meal go, however, until probiotics have a chance to eke a bit more nutritional value from what's left. Probiotics break some kinds of fiber into short-chain fatty acids such as butyrate, which is then directly utilized as fuel by the cells that line the colon wall.

Cholesterol that ends up in the colon is used to make steroid hormones, which can then pass through the walls of the colon back into the circulation. This can have the effect of lowering circulating levels of cholesterol—a good thing, considering that more than 13 million Americans are on cholesterol-lowering statin drugs!

Estrogen levels in the body are also affected by the type and number of colon bacteria. When probiotic enzyme activity decreases, blood levels of estrogen also decrease—possibly indicating a relationship between colon dysbiosis and diseases that involve estrogen, including osteoporosis and breast cancer.

The Perils of Dysbiosis

When your diet is rich in fiber and fluids and your gastrointestinal physiology is otherwise in balance, the resulting stools are soft (but not too soft) and are easily passed. If internal ecology is not in equilibrium, the result can be constipation—where stools stay too long in the colon, making them hard and difficult to pass—or diarrhea, where unfriendly bacteria stimulate the colon to get rid of its contents before enough water or electrolytes can be reabsorbed. Insufficient probiotic populations in the colon also contribute to gas, flatulence, and bloating.

All of these symptoms are typical of irritable bowel syndrome (IBS), a disorder that mainstream medicine has not been able to explain or treat effectively with drugs. Alternative practitioners, on the other hand, have successfully treated IBS with natural protocols that include probiotic supplements. Now that the majority of research into IBS and probiotics suppports this approach, the medical mainstream is beginning to change its tune and employ good bacteria in the fight against this unpleasant malady.

Probiotics for Diarrhea

Diarrhea is undeniably an uncomfortable problem, but it almost always strikes for good reason. It is your body's way of quickly moving harmful substances—including foods that don't agree with you, or pathogenic bacteria—out of your body. When the immune cells that line the intestinal tract perceive a threat in something you've eaten or that has passed into your intestines through a leaky gut wall, the muscles that line the small and large intestines shift into overdrive, contracting powerfully to move the threatening substance out before it can adhere to the intestinal wall or be absorbed. This happens so quickly that there's no time for the reabsorption of water and electrolytes in the colon, and so the bowel movements that result are watery.

Crohn's Disease

A chronic inflammatory disease that can affect any part of the GI tract. Symptoms include pain, fever, diarrhea, and weight loss.

Drugs for diarrhea typically work by slowing intestinal contractions or by solidifying stools. These approaches may deal with the immediate problem, but they set you up for more long-term problems by retaining pathogens or other toxic substances inside your body. A better approach is to improve the body's ability to deal with those substances, and probiotics are a good way to accomplish this end.

Diarrhea is one of the more troublesome symptoms of inflammatory bowel disease (including Crohn's disease and ulcerative colitis) and irritable bowel syndrome (IBS). Many sufferers of these often painful maladies, for which mainstream medicine has no lasting solutions, turn to drugs that can do more harm than good: steroids such as Prednisone are sometimes effective, but don't cure these diseases.

Ulcerative Colitis
Chronic inflammation and ulceration of the lining of the colon and rectum. Symptoms include bloody diarrhea, fever, abdominal pain, and feelings of unwellness.

Crohn's and ulcerative colitis sufferers are believed to have twenty times the likelihood of developing colon cancer compared to those without these inflammatory gastrointestinal conditions.

Irritable bowel syndrome—also known as "spastic colon"—consists of a poorly understood group of symptoms, including abdominal pain, flatulence, bloating, and irregular bowel movements. Ten to 20 percent of adults in the United States have at least some of these symptoms on a regular basis; 25 to 50 percent of those who visit a gastroenterologist's office do so because of symptoms suggestive of IBS. Some people with IBS are chronically constipated; others have chronic diarrhea; still others have episodes of both. Several studies have shown that IBS sufferers have abnormal gut bacteria. In one such study, researchers found that subjects with IBS had lower numbers of lactobacilli and bifidobacteria compared to healthy controls.

Probiotics have been shown to benefit IBS patients. For example, in one Swedish study, published in the *American Journal of Gastroenterology*, sixty IBS patients were given the probiotic *L. plantarum* for four weeks. Their gas and pain were significantly reduced and their overall gastrointestinal function improved. In another study, researchers showed that probiotic supplementation gave IBS sufferers pronounced relief within two weeks of the beginning of the study. Another research team showed that the gut bacteria of twenty IBS patients were of similar composition, with decreased lactobacilli and bifidobacteria compared to healthy controls.

University of Alberta professor Richard N. Fedorak, M.D., is an expert on inflammatory bowel disease (IBD). According to his research, IBD is caused by the passage of pathogenic bacteria, or a toxin produced by those bacteria, into the intestines. They may adhere to the intestinal lining. In most people, this elicits an immune response in the intestines that handles the problem. Those who suffer from IBD, however, have genetic traits that cause the immune cells that line the intestines to overreact to the pathogen, creating inflammation that ends up injuring the intestinal lining and causing IBD symptoms.

Probiotics protect against IBD by adhering to the intestinal lining and preventing the adhesion or crossing-over of harmful bacteria. Friendly bacteria can actually move through already-adhered layers of harmful bugs to offer this protection. Additional studies from Dr. Fedorak's laboratory have shown reduced counts of bifidobacteria in fecal and tissue samples of Crohn's disease and reduced counts of *Lactobacillus* in ulcerative colitis; the worse the symptoms, the lower the numbers of these good bugs. Researchers at UNC Chapel Hill found that therapy with *Lactobacillus rhamnosus* prevented the relapse of colitis in rats, and that *L. plantarum* prevents and treats colitis in mice.

Probiotic supplementation also benefits viral diarrhea. It has been found to decrease viral shedding and increase secretory IgA, an antibody associated with improved healing from viral infection.

Diarrhea Caused by Antibiotics

A bad case of diarrhea often follows a course of antibiotics. In hospital settings, such diarrhea is often caused by virulent bacteria called *Clostridium*. This infection—which can cause colitis, toxic megacolon (a severe condition that requires surgical removal of part of or all of the large intestine), even death—only becomes established in a colon with imbalanced microflora.

Much of the research that is most supportive of probiotic supplementation has dealt with antibiotic-associated diarrhea. In fact, probiotics have been used for this purpose since the 1950s. An analysis of nine studies on this subject found that *Lactobacilli* worked significantly better than placebo for the prevention of this type of diarrhea. Live-culture yogurt has been found in several studies to prevent or decrease the duration of antibiotic-associated diarrhea. Bacterial strains that have been found to help heal or prevent antibiotic-related diarrhea include:

- *Lactobacillus rhamnosus*
- *Lactobacillus acidophilus*

- *Bifidobacterium longum*
- *Enterococcus faecium*

Antibiotic therapy can also cause yeast overgrowth by killing off probiotics and allowing yeasts to grow out of control. This is why vaginal yeast infection is common in the aftermath of a course of antibiotics. If you need to take antibiotic drugs, take a quality probiotic supplement (I'll tell you how to choose one in Chapter 9) between antibiotic doses, and continue to do so following antibiotic therapy.

Traveler's Diarrhea

Overseas travel can lead to a condition inelegantly known as "traveler's trots"—a type of diarrhea caused by exposure to non-pathogenic but unfamiliar bacteria. Research from Guatemala, Nepal, and Mexico has shown that travelers who take probiotics fare much better than those who don't when it comes to this condition, which can all but ruin a dream vacation. If you take an adequate dose of probiotics every day for a week before leaving on your overseas voyage and continue to do so throughout the trip, your likelihood of developing traveler's diarrhea will fall dramatically.

Probiotic bacteria plays multiple roles in the maintenance of a healthy large intestine, showing promise as a preventative and treatment for diarrhea, constipation, irritable bowel syndrome, inflammatory bowel disease, and colon cancer. Optimal health can't be achieved without colon health; it's just that simple.

CHAPTER 4

PROBIOTICS AND IMMUNE SYSTEM SUPPORT

The immune system employs an incredibly complex and highly effective set of defenses and offenses against pathogens and antigens. From the time a new person enters the world, his or her body begins to build its resistance against whatever microbes it might happen to encounter. Antibodies, cytokines, macrophages, phagocytes, and numerous other types of immune cells and substances are continually created to protect us against disease-causing organisms. These cells are produced by the bone marrow, thymus, and spleen.

Pathogen
Any agent (particularly, any microorganism) that causes disease.

Antigen
Any agent that stimulates the immune system to form antibodies.

Today, worries about once life-threatening infections have dwindled because of antibiotics and other drugs, better hospitals, and better overall hygiene: plentiful food, clean drinking water, adequate systems for disposing of wastes, and clean environments in which to live. We have vaccines for several diseases that once caused considerable problems, especially in children. The catch here is that today's immune systems—those of humans who live in developed nations—are being altered for the worse by frequent use of antibiotics and overzealous use of vaccinations. As a result, immune dysfunction is far more common than it should be, given the relative wealth and easy access to medical care enjoyed by most who live in first world nations.

Defects in immune function can have catastrophic consequences. I'm not just talking about immunity that isn't up to par, either; remember the Bubble Boy, who had to live in a sealed plastic room to avoid contact with pathogens? I'm also talking about *overactive* immunity, the kind that attacks its host in the form of allergies, asthma, and autoimmune disease. Cancerous cells exist in every person's body. Under the best of circumstances, our immune systems are able to target and eliminate them before they have a chance to spread. When immune function isn't up to par, cancer cells are more likely to take hold.

Probiotics have documented balancing effects on the immune system, and have long been believed to assist in the fight against cancer. Most of the research into immune effects of friendly bacteria is done using fermented milk, which you and I know as yogurt. Some theorize that substances released from the milk during fermentation have immune-enhancing properties.

Probiotics Reduce the Need for Antibiotics

The overuse of antibiotics is a worrisome problem. For decades, they have been prescribed to patients who don't really need them, and on top of this they're loaded into livestock to enhance their growth and weight gain. To put it mildly, we are chronically overexposed to bacteria-busting drugs, and our immune systems are suffering as antibiotic-resistant bugs gear up to take over the world.

Antibiotic drugs kill off bacteria both good and bad. Once the drug is stopped, the dearth of good bugs gives any antibiotic-resistant bad bugs that remain *carte blanche*. These opportunistic organisms multiply unfettered by the good bacteria cops that usually patrol the intestines, and the result can be diarrhea or severe gastrointestinal infections.

The World Health Organization (WHO) has recommended that antibiotics in medical practice and livestock need to be cut back dramatically. Now that the problems with antibiotic overuse are becoming common knowledge, doctors are finally beginning to prescribe them less. They'd do a lot better to also prescribe probiotic therapy to people who are fighting infection, particularly infections that affect the GI tract or mucous membranes, including the bladder, urinary tract, vaginal tract, and respiratory tract. In 1994, the World Health Organization recommended the use of probiotics as second-line therapy when antibiotics don't work.

Probiotics defend against pathogenic bacteria in several ways. They compete for nutrients, regulate the immune system, and increase the activity of genes in the gut that are associated with improved resistance against unfriendly bugs. They also lower colon pH, which creates an environment that's comfortable for probiotics and uncomfortable for harmful yeasts, molds, and bacteria.

One of the best tactics employed in our defense by probiotics is the production of antitoxins—substances that inhibit the growth of their less friendly competitors and protect against the toxins they give off. *L. acidophilus* (DDS-1 strain) produces acidophilin, a bacteria-killing substance that is known to have antibiotic effects against at least twenty-two other strains of bacteria, including *E. coli, Shigella dysenteriae, Staphylococcus aureus, Streptococcus lactis, Klebsiella pneumoniae,* and *Salmonella schottmuelleri.* Cancer research over the past decade has found that *E. coli* in the intestines synthesizes carcinogenic chemicals (nitrosamine and ethionine). Probiotics are nature's way of controlling this bacterial threat.

Other substances made by probiotics can inhibit the growth of *H. pylori,* the bacteria that indirectly causes ulcers to form and increases stomach cancer risk.

Enhancement of White Blood Cell Activity

White blood cells actually describes a class of immune cells that includes neutrophils, eosinophils, basophils, monocytes, macrophages, and lymphocytes. They are produced by B cells and T cells and defend against the invasion of foreign microbes in two ways: by creating inflammation, and by literally engulfing and digesting organisms tagged as potentially harmful. Probiotics enhance the ability of white blood cells (also known as phagocytes) to engulf and digest pathogens.

Inflammation

Crucial element of the immune response that creates heat, swelling, and pain at the location of infection or trauma.

Animals that are fed fermented milk show increases in the activity of both phagocytes and lymphocytes within three days. Macrophage activity also rises in response to probiotic supplementation. A study performed at the Université de Moncton in Canada found that regular feedings of milk fermented with *Lactobacillus helveticus* enhanced the activity of macrophages in the GI tracts of mice within a week. Another study, this one from Australian researchers, found that four common *Lactobacillus* strains increased lymphocyte production.

Enhanced Antibody Production

Antibodies are specialized proteins produced by immune cells called B cells. The B cells are responsible for identifying potentially dangerous antigens; once they've done so, they "tag" the antigen with an antibody. This is the immunological equivalent of a bullseye. Once an antibody is present, other types of immune cells target it for destruction.

Vaccines work by introducing enough of an altered version of a microorganism to elicit an antibody response, but not enough to actually cause the disease. As soon as you're exposed to a microorganism you've been vaccinated against, your body starts to make antibodies to it, and theoretically, it doesn't stand a chance. Antibodies are grouped into separate categories: IgA, IgG, IgM, and IgD. ("Ig" stands for *immunoglobulin*.)

Animal and test tube studies have shown that probiotics enhance the body's ability to produce IgA and IgG antibodies. *Lactobacillus* was found to improve the body's production of IgM in response to a rotavirus vaccine, and another study found that antibody response to a typhoid vaccination was improved with the same probiotic bacteria. This effect of probiotics likely has to do with increased binding of both good and bad bugs to the intestinal lining, which activates antibody production there.

Improved antibody production means you'll get sick less, because your body will be able to target and eliminate illness-causing bugs before they can take hold.

Good Bacteria Help Immune Cells Talk to One Another

Probiotics also enhance the production of *cytokines*, which are hormone-like messengers immune cells use to communicate with each other. Subtle changes in cytokine production are interpreted by the immune system, which then changes its activity accordingly, mobilizing certain kinds of immune cells to crack down on pathogens. *Interleukins* are a particularly intriguing variety of cytokine; they communicate with both immune cells and cells of the nervous system. This could be the link between immunity and thoughts and emotions—one reason why having a stressful week might make you succumb to a cold; why being sick can have such intense emotional repercussions; and why visualization of immune system "good guys" attacking cancer cells has the effect of amping up immune defenses against cancer.

Cytokines play a crucial role in maintaining a balanced immune system. Immune deficits can be a problem, but so can an immune system that doesn't know when to say when. Certain types of cytokines send out a message to cool it when the awesome power of the immune system threatens to injure its host, such as interleukin-10 (IL-10). Probiotics have been found to promote the activity of IL-10.

Resist Allergies, Asthma, and Eczema with Probiotics

Inflammation is a necessary part of normal immune response, but in certain people inflammation gets out of control and creates the runny nose and itchy eyes of allergies, the bronchial swelling and mucus production of asthma, the itchy rash of eczema, or other manifestations of allergy.

Probiotics have the amazing ability to stimulate immune function in those who are lacking and to down-regulate inflammatory responses in those who tend toward hypersensitivity. In one study by a well-known probiotics researcher, it was found that people with milk allergy (not to be confused with lactose intolerance) respond to probiotic supplementation with immune changes that reflect decreased inflammation; subjects without milk allergy got an immune system boost from the same probiotic.

People who have allergies, asthma, and eczema are more likely than others to suffer from leaky gut and food allergies. Their bodies are in a constant state of low-grade inflammation, which can manifest itself as runny nose, itchy eyes, swollen airways, itchy, flaky skin, or other allergic symptoms. As you've already learned, probiotics are a major part of any program for healing leaky gut and decreasing overzealous gut inflammation. According to studies performed on animal models, probiotics may even help digest allergens before they can affect the gut wall or move into the bloodstream.

Some of the most promising research into the anti-allergy and anti-eczema effects of probiotics deal with infants and children. I'll tell you more about this in Chapter 7. For example, in infants who had developed eczema, a one-month trial supplementation of *Lactobacillus* significantly improved their condition.

In infants with already established eczema, significant improvements in dermatitis were noted after a one-month trial with *Lactobacillus* fortified hydrolyzed whey formula. The authors of the study suggest that "probiotics may enhance endogenous barrier mechanisms of the gut and alleviate intestinal inflammation, providing a useful tool for treating food allergy."

Autoimmune Disease May Be Caused by Dysbiosis

Indirect effects of probiotics on autoimmune processes, likely mediated by changes in inflammatory mediators, (e.g., cytokines) may be related to regulation or modulation of the immune system, both locally in the GI tract and systemically.

The intestines contain a higher concentration of immune cells than any other organ. This makes sense when you consider that the intestinal wall has to protect against every single pathogenic substance that enters our bodies in the foods we eat, the drugs we swallow, and whatever else might accidentally find its way into the gut.

Good bacteria are particularly effective at modulating what is known as the *gut immune system*, the various immune components that live and work within the walls of the intestines. When these bacteria are not present in adequate numbers, or when more dangerous bugs overtake them, a state of dysbiosis sets in.

Dysbiosis has far-reaching effects on the immune system. Nearly a century's worth of research has shown that people with rheumatoid arthritis have immune complexes from unfriendly gut bacteria in their bloodstreams. It's likely that a combination of leaky gut and dysbiosis conspire to create harmful inflammatory processes in the body; in the case of rheumatoid arthritis, inflammation settles into the joints, but can also affect the organs. Treatment with fasting, vegan diets, and reinoculation with beneficial bacteria and the foods that support them has shown far more promise than mainstream therapies, which involve dangerous chemotherapy drugs such as methotrexate and the risky newer medicine, Enbrel.

In a study of thirty children with chronic juvenile arthritis—a type of arthritis that causes painful inflammation in the joints—*Lactobacillus* was given for two weeks. The researchers kept close track of changes in the gut immune system and other measures of gut health throughout the study's duration. In the end, it was concluded that gut defenses are disturbed in children with chronic juvenile arthritis, and that these disturbances cause inflammation and increase intestinal permeability (leaky gut). The study's results make a good case for therapy with probiotics in children, and by association, in adults with rheumatoid arthritis.

Probiotics reduce fecal urease, an enzyme that is associated with chronic arthritic inflammation. In a study conducted by Irish researchers and presented at Digestive Disease Week 2000, it was discovered that

Lactobacillus salivarius helped to inhibit the production of inflammatory cytokines such as TNF-alpha in the intestinal lining.

This study also examined the balance of Th2 and Th1 responses. "Th" stands for "T helper," and the Th1 cells help cell-killing, inflammation-producing T cells while the Th2 cells help antibody-making B cells. The balance of Th1 and Th2 is an excellent indicator of the immune system's ability to mount attacks against dangerous pathogens without overdoing it and causing allergic or autoimmune problems. Several strains of *Lactobacillus* appear to be capable of enhancing Th2 (antibody-making) response and suppressing inflammatory Th1 response.

Probiotics Help Resist Cancer Initiation and Growth

Modern humans are constantly exposed to vast numbers of synthetic chemical toxins, many of which are suspected or known carcinogens. Never before has it been so important to optimize our bodies' ability to defuse carcinogenic threats. Fortunately, probiotics can play a role in doing just that. Studies in test tubes and on animals have revealed that probiotics can inhibit the growth of cancerous tumors induced by toxic chemicals.

In order for cancer to take root and grow, it must undergo two distinct stages. First, there's *initiation,* where a non-cancerous cell is transformed into a cancerous one. This can happen as a result of exposure to toxins that alter cells' genetic codes, or heredity, or excessive free radical formation, or a combination of these and other factors. Once initiation has taken place, *progression*—the multiplication and spread of cancer—is the next step. Sometimes progression happens rapidly, and sometimes it happens slowly or not at all.

Probiotics can stop cancer before it starts by inhibiting the action of substances that cause cells to become cancerous. Strong evidence supports the theory that dysbiosis plays a role in causing gastrointestinal cancers. Most carcinogenic substances that enter the body in foods we eat aren't carcinogenic when we swallow them. The activity of enzymes throughout the GI tract and in the liver alters these substances in ways that bring out their cancer-causing potential. A healthful balance of good and bad bacteria in the digestive tract creates an enzymatic environment that helps to prevent the formation of carcinogens; when bad bacteria begin to overtake the good, more of the enzymes that create carcinogens are produced.

L. acidophilus (DDS-1), *L. bulgaricus,* and *S. thermophilus* have direct antitumor effects. Fermented milk has been found to slow the proliferation of breast cancer cells in laboratory studies. Researchers have found that they can reduce cancer cell formation in the colon. *Bifidobacteria* directly inhibit the activity of less friendly bowel bacteria that transform nitrates, which are commonly found in processed foods, into carcinogenic nitrites. In two studies of yogurt consumption's effects on experimental colon cancer, test animals that were fed yogurt while being exposed to a potent carcinogen showed increased *apoptosis.* Increases in cancer-fighting interleukins and cytokines were also found in one of these studies.

In another study, this one by scientists at the American Health Foundation in Valhalla, New York, the effects of *prebiotics* (the preferred foods of probiotics) on cancer growth was evaluated. The researchers fed lab rats oligofructose and inulin, both of which stimulate the growth of bifidobacteria.

> **Apoptosis**
>
> *Programmed cell death. Healthy cells are programmed to die, so they can be replaced by new cells. When apoptosis is turned off, the door is opened to uncontrolled cell growth—cancer.*

The prebiotics inhibited the growth of precancerous colon lesions. Earlier studies in the same laboratory found that encouraging *Bifidobacteria* growth also inhibits the growth of chemically induced breast cancer.

Radiation Therapy and Probiotics

Conventional cancer treatment often involves the use of targeted radiation. Radiation can do a lot to shrink tumors and stunt their growth, but it does so at a significant price. Skin burns and disturbances in intestinal microflora are among the side effects of radiation therapy. Pelvic radiotherapy is the worst culprit when it comes to killing off friendly flora, making way for pathogenic bacteria that end up causing severe inflammation and leaky gut. It's no surprise that diarrhea and intestinal infections are common side effects of radiotherapy.

The daily consumption of probiotic-containing yogurt or use of probiotic supplements before, during, and after radiotherapy can help you get through this toxic treatment with your GI system still in good working order.

Cancer is probably the most feared disease of our time. If maintaining a balanced internal ecosystem can help us to avoid a cancer diagnosis—in addition to all the other benefits of probiotics—it certainly seems worth the effort.

CHAPTER 5

PROBIOTICS FOR REPRODUCTIVE AND URINARY TRACT HEALTH

Disorders of the urinary tract and vaginal tract affect an estimated 1 billion women per year. The most common of these are bacterial vaginosis (BV), vaginal yeast infection (yeast vaginitis), and urinary tract infection (UTI). Mainstream medicine offers both oral and topical medications to deal with these problems, and for the most part, they work, at least temporarily. They don't deal with the underlying imbalances that create these illnesses, however, and in some cases, they actually aggravate those imbalances.

Let's take vaginal yeast infections, for example. When a woman takes a course of antibiotics, *Candida* yeast can grow unfettered because the probiotics that normally police the body have been eradicated. The result is often a yeast infection. Now, let's say that infection is treated with the usual course of antifungal drugs, such as fluconazole, clotrimazole, ketoconazole, or itraconazole. If you're treating a vaginal bacterial infection, you'll probably be told to take antibiotics or use intravaginal antibiotics, which will set you up for—you guessed it—vaginal yeast infection! It's a no-win situation.

Even if these scenarios don't happen, the antifungal and antibiotic drugs used to treat BV, UTI, and vaginal yeast infection have potential side effects that are best avoided if at all possible. By this point you understand why antibiotics are a bad idea unless absolutely necessary. Antifungal drugs interact dangerously with a long list of other drugs, and these interactions can happen even when antifungals are used intravaginally rather than orally.

Probiotics to the Rescue

Friendly bacteria colonize both the vaginal and urinary tracts. Most of the bacteria that end up populating the vagina are *Lactobacillus*, which produce both lactic acid and hydrogen peroxide in quantities sufficient to hamper the growth of pathogens.

Modulating the intestinal microflora with oral probiotic supplements alters the probiotic strains found in both the vagina and the urinary tract. This is a natural consequence of the close proximity of the openings of both of these organs to the opening at the termination of the large intestine (less delicately known as the anus), as well as enhancing immune function in both of these organs. By maintaining the integrity of the intestinal wall and preventing infection or excessive inflammation from taking hold there, probiotics enhance the body's overall resistance to infection.

As you might have guessed, probiotics are useful for bacterial vaginosis, which is really a sign that vaginal flora have fallen out of balance. Probiotics can also be used—along with other natural therapies—to treat urinary tract infection and yeast infection. This is true even if you need to augment treatment with mainstream medications. Do not use probiotics and antibiotics at the same time.

Treating Bacterial Vaginosis (BV) with Probiotics

It's believed that 30 to 50 percent of women of reproductive age have BV, making it the primary cause of abnormal vaginal discharge. Half of these women have no symptoms. Left untreated, bacterial vaginosis can cause infertility, pelvic infection, and ectopic pregancy. Fifteen to 25 percent of pregnant women have some form of BV, and this disorder is known to drastically increase risk of low birth weight, prematurity, and premature rupture of membranes (PROM).

What causes BV? First and foremost, there are the factors that lower probiotic populations throughout the body: antibiotics, poor diet, stress, and the other factors that are listed in the Introduction. BV is *not* a sexually transmitted disease, although women who have more frequent sex are more likely to have it. Douching, which throws vaginal flora out of balance, can also cause BV.

Whether or not a woman requires antibiotic therapy, probiotics can be used to reestablish

Bacterial Vaginosis (BV)

An overgrowth of pathogenic bacteria that normally reside in the vagina, causing a thin whitish discharge, a fishy odor, itching, or no symptoms at all.

healthy vaginal flora. If you're a woman treating BV, and you aren't having uncomfortable symptoms, you might try probiotics alone first to give your body an opportunity to knock out the infection on its own. This is an especially good idea for pregnant women who don't want to expose their growing babies to antibiotics. Check with your doctor for a firm diagnosis and make sure you're safe putting off the antibiotics for a few days.

Lactobacilli use a few tactics to keep vaginal infection at bay. First, they create an inhospitable environment by secreting hydrogen peroxide and acids. If this doesn't work and pathogens begin to multiply, they block the adhesion of those pathogens to vaginal tissues; if this doesn't forestall the infection, lactobacilli begin to target and eliminate infectious organisms that have infiltrated the cells of the vaginal lining. A study published in the *Journal of Infectious Disease* in 2001 evaluated the ability of lactobacilli to block the colonization of pathogenic bacteria in the cells of the vaginal lining. The researchers found that the growth of these pathogens was blocked by 50 to 74 percent.

Take an oral probiotic supplement and try a douche made of *Lactobacillus*-containing yogurt each night before bed for a few days. Or, if you'd like a less messy option, open up a probiotic capsule and sprinkle its contents on a moistened tampon. Insert the tampon overnight, and do so for a few consecutive nights.

Vaginal *L. acidophilus* tablets may soon be available. One group of researchers administered a vaginal tablet containing this friendly bacteria along with 0.03 mg of estriol (a type of estrogen). The study involved thirty-two women with BV, some of whom received one to two tablets a day and the rest of whom received a placebo treatment. Two weeks later, 77 percent of the women in the treatment group were cured, and only 25 percent of the control group enjoyed the same results. The strains used were shown to effectively colonize the vaginal tissues. In another study, researchers gave twenty-eight women with BV a probiotic suppository, and gave twenty-nine BV sufferers a placebo. By the end of six days, sixteen of the twenty-eight probiotic users no longer had BV. None of the placebo patients was cured during that six-day span.

Most of the women in this study's treatment group had a recurrence following their next period—a sign that longer treatment might have been necessary. Some probiotic bacteria adhere and colonize better than others; those that don't readily take up residence within the body can still protect against pathogens, as long as they are taken on a daily basis. Some experts advise that supplemental versions be used continuously long-term—(for weeks or months) to continually correct vaginal pH.

Knock Out Vaginal Yeast Infections with Probiotics

Often women with bacterial vaginosis mistakenly believe that they're dealing with a yeast infection. They treat themselves with over-the-counter yeast infection treatments, and these antifungal drugs won't do a thing for BV. Some women have both problems at once—not surprising, when you consider that they both spring from imbalances between good and bad bacteria. If you have been trying without luck to cure what you believe to be a chronic yeast infection, see your OB/GYN to be tested for bacterial vaginosis.

Vaginal Yeast Infection

An overgrowth of Candida yeast in the vagina, causing thick whitish discharge, a yeasty odor, itching, and irritation.

Of course, you could also try treating yourself with probiotics. Unlike antifungals or antibiotics, probiotics deal with both BV and vaginal yeast at their source: unbalanced vaginal flora. In 1992, the first rigorously performed clinical study on this subject showed that when women eat yogurt fermented with live *L. acidophilus* culture, they are decreasing the ability of candida to colonize the vagina and cause yeast infection. A study published in 1996 showed that eating yogurt with *L. acidophilus* helped a significant number of women to get rid of both vaginal yeast infection and BV.

Urinary Tract Infection (UTI):
A Sign That Probiotics Are Needed

Urinary tract infection causes pain, burning, and a sensation of constantly having to urinate. They're often recurrent and can lead to kidney infection if not promptly treated. Women are more vulnerable to UTI than men, probably because their urinary tract openings are so close to other openings that can harbor pathogenic bacteria. In fact, the pathogenic bacteria that most commonly cause UTI are those found in the feces.

Urinary Tract Infection

Overgrowth of pathogenic bacteria in the urinary tract; commonly occurs in women with BV or vaginal yeast overgrowth.

Finnish researchers set out to discover whether altering intestinal flora with live-culture yogurt would help to prevent UTI in 139 healthy college-aged women. They gathered dietary information on their subjects and found that women who ate the most fermented milk products and freshly squeezed juices—particularly juices made from berries—were a bit more than half as likely to have a UTI during the course of the study. Interestingly, women in this study who had intercourse more often (three or more times a week versus one or less times a week) were almost three times as likely to end up with a UTI. Spermicide use has also been linked with increased UTI risk.

Although the link between UTI and shortage of probiotics isn't as clear as the link between good bacteria and vaginal infection, all the evidence points to the helpful role probiotics can play in preventing and treating this often chronic problem. Both oral and vaginal probiotic suppositories have been shown to be effective at reducing recurrent UTI incidence.

If you are prone to UTIs, also keep in mind that cranberries contain phytochemicals (plant chemicals) that inhibit the adhesion of bad bacteria to the walls of the urinary tract. As soon as you feel a UTI coming on, start drinking cranberry juice (not cranberry juice cocktail, but the real, tart, unsweetened variety) or take a cranberry extract. Be sure to drink lots and lots of water, as well.

Hygiene is an important factor in prevention of UTI and BV. Always wipe from front to back after a bowel movement. Urinating right after intercourse will also help to keep the urinary tract healthy. Spermicides are best avoided by women who are prone to UTIs; choose a form of birth control that doesn't require them.

Vaginal and urinary tract health are inextricably tied to microflora balance. Anyone who is prone to either type of problem—and most who tend toward one also tend toward the other, because the causes are so similar—would do well to take the necessary steps to balance her internal ecosystem.

CHAPTER 6

BETTER SKIN
WITH PROBIOTICS

Skin problems are almost always more than skin deep. When you break out in a rash, hives, or acne lesions, you're getting a sign from within your body that something is out of balance. This is why skin creams or topical medications usually don't fix the problem, at least not more than temporarily.

Some skin problems, such as dermatitis, eczema, and psoriasis, are allergic in nature. Acne is an inflammation of the sweat glands and/ or hair follicles that causes blackheads, whiteheads, pustules ("zits" or "pimples"), nodules (firm swellings beneath the skin), and cysts (larger swellings). Both types of skin disorders can be helped with the appropriate use of probiotics.

The Role of Good Bacteria in Skin Health

Both good and bad bacteria can be found on the skin's surface and within its tissues. Skin provides a barrier that safeguards internal organs against contact with pathogens, but it's more than a simple wall to those destructive bugs; immune cells are highly active all along those borders. Think of the good skin bacteria as the troops along the borders of an already well-fortified territory, preventing enemy troops from ever marshalling a serious effort to invade and take over.

Maintaining good bacteria in the GI tract aids in the absorption of nutrients and helps to prevent the absorption of allergenic substances. Without adequate nutrients, skin cells can't do the work necessary to keep your exterior surfaces healthy and smooth.

Naturopathic medicine holds that skin diseases are signs that toxicity from inside the body is trying to find its way out through the skin, and that these toxins cause inflammation and irritation as they move out of the body. Colonic flora help to remove toxins as they pass through the GI tract, so that they aren't reabsorbed through the colon wall to be excreted through the skin.

Probiotics and Acne

Hormone imbalances—especially those characteristic of the teen years—cause sebum to be overproduced within the sebaceous glands. The follicle gets clogged, and pathogenic bacteria begin to build up, causing inflammation.

Sebum

Oily fluid made within sebaceous glands to lubricate the skin and flush dead cells out of the hair follicles.

Acne is probably the most common skin-related complaint, affecting about 75 percent of all Americans at some time between the ages of twelve and twenty-four. So-called adult acne affects many people at thirty, forty, and beyond. Mainstream therapy includes both topical treatments (benzoyl peroxide, retinoic acid, antibiotic lotions, sulfur-based creams) and antibiotics such as tetracycline. Topical therapies don't do much more than aid in the healing of acne once it's developed. Long-term antibiotic therapy has the effect of killing off good bacteria and is likely to give rise to antibiotic-resistant bacteria that continue to cause acne lesions.

In the mid-1960s, physician R. H. Siver was conducting a study of probiotics as therapy for stomach and intestinal problems. As he tracked the progress of his subjects, he noticed an interesting side effect of probiotic therapy: facial acne cleared in 80 percent of those who had been suffering from it, within two weeks in most cases. A study by Italian researchers also shows that balancing of intestinal flora may be an important missing link in current acne therapy.

Allergic Skin Disorders and Probiotics

Allergic skin problems cause itchy, bumpy, often unsightly rashes that crop up and disappear for no apparent reason. *Dermatitis* and *eczema* are terms that are often used interchangeably to describe allergic skin problems; from here on, I'll refer to these problems as eczema. The tendency to develop eczema is greater in people whose relatives have had a tendency toward allergy. It's quite common for eczema sufferers to also suffer from allergic rhinitis (nasal allergy) and/or asthma. Food allergy is an important cause of eczema; elimination diets have been found to help a significant portion of those who suffer from this sometimes disfiguring skin problem.

Babies and young children seem especially susceptible to eczema. Ninety percent of those who suffer from eczema are under the age of five; six percent are between ages six and ten, with only 2 percent of people aged ten and up suffering from the same complaint. This is likely due to the relative immaturity of the gastrointestinal tracts of infants and young children—immaturity that makes them more susceptible to developing leaky gut when allergenic foods are eaten. The average American child eats almost nothing *but* allergenic foods, with white flour and dairy for almost every meal, and tends not to eat foods that foster the growth of good bacteria.

Often, the only mainstream therapy that works for allergic skin disease sufferers are cortisone-based skin creams, which soothe symptoms temporarily but only work as long as they're used. Long-term application of steroid creams to the skin isn't recommended; even the small amounts that soak into the body can have suppressant effects on the body's own production of the important hormone cortisol. Interestingly, a link has been identified between the suppression of the inflammation that causes the redness, itching, and blistering of eczema with steroid creams and the worsening of asthma.

A good deal of research has been done to discern whether probiotic therapy could help those with eczema. It makes sense that friendly bacteria would have this effect, considering the fact that they do so much to control leaky gut. Studies have demonstrated that children with a tendency to develop allergies (including eczema) have imbalanced intestinal microflora and increased intestinal permeability. Probiotics normalize intestinal permeability, improve the gut's immunological defense barrier, and tone down intestinal immune response.

In one study by a research team from Denmark, children aged between one and ten took either a probiotic supplement (containing *Lactobacillus rhamnosus* and *Lactobacillus reuteri*) or a placebo each day for six weeks. At the study's conclusion, 56 percent of the children who took the *Lactobacillus* experienced significant improvement, while only 15 percent of the children on placebo had similar improvements. Another study, this one from Finland, looked at the production of an anti-inflammatory interleukin, IL-10, in children with eczema who were given *L. rhamnosus*. After eight weeks, blood samples showed enhanced IL-10 generation. Other research shows that administration of probiotics to infants cut the incidence of eczema before age two in half; a follow-up study by the same research group found that this protection lasted through the childrens' fourth birthdays.

University of Turku's Department of Pediatrics in Finland gave *Lactobacillus* to pregnant women who had at least one first-degree relative or partner with nasal allergies, asthma, or eczema, and then gave the same probiotic to their infants for the first six months postpartum. Only fourteen of the fifty-three children who received the probiotic developed eczema, compared with twenty-five of the fifty-four on placebo.

Most of the research on eczema and probiotics has been done with children, because they are most likely to suffer from the disease. There's no reason to believe, however, that the same tactics found to be successful with children wouldn't be useful for adults who continue to battle this itchy, uncomfortable problem. The use of probiotics for other allergic skin diseases such as psoriasis and acne rosacea has been less well researched; still, when you consider the mechanisms by which probiotics heal the gut and prevent allergens from moving into the bloodstream to affect immune cells in the skin, it makes sense to add these good bugs to your optimal health program if you have any kind of allergic condition at all.

Eczema Control and Food Allergy Control Go Hand in Hand

Although probiotics will help you to control eczema, you'll need to identify and eliminate allergenic foods from your diet to finish the job. It's not easy, but the payoff is great. Not only will you experience relief from eczema, you'll also get relief from nasal allergies and asthma—which, as an eczema sufferer, you're more likely to have than the general population.

Start your elimination diet by continuing to eat normally for a week, carefully recording everything you eat in a food diary. At week's end, go through the record and identify the foods you ate at every meal or almost every meal. Then, identify the basic ingredients in those foods and eliminate them completely from your diet for six weeks. For example, bread, cereal, and pasta are all comprised mostly of wheat, while cheese, milk, and ice cream are all categorized as dairy. Wheat and dairy are the most common allergenic foods.

Be sure to carefully eliminate all sources of the foods you eat daily or almost daily. Processed foods often contain hidden ingredients that make this practice difficult, so stick with unadulterated whole foods—whole grains, vegetables, fruit, and lean protein—while you're on this diet, and take a probiotic supplement (non-dairy if you are off dairy). You can also use the amino acid glutamine to enhance the healing of leaky gut; try 500 mg twice a day.

Keep track of symptoms throughout your diet. You may find you're feeling so much better that you'll want to continue this diet indefinitely. After six weeks, you can probably go back to eating small amounts of the foods you're sensitive to, but only do so two or three times a week; otherwise, you'll end up right back where you started.

CHAPTER 7

PROBIOTICS AND CHILDREN'S HEALTH

As a baby passes through its mother's birth canal, it is exposed to the health-promoting bacteria that populate its mother's vagina. This is Mother Nature's way of introducing these good bugs to the newborn's intestinal tract. Today, about 20 percent of babies are born by Cesarean section in the United States, and this practice brings many infants into the world without this important first dose of probiotics. This explains why babies born by C-section tend to have more gastrointestinal issues than babies born vaginally.

In developed nations, unfortunately, there's an increasing trend toward elective C-section. Aside from the probiotic dose a vaginally born infant gets, there are a lot of reasons why C-section should only be performed when absolutely necessary. While natural childbirth is not exactly a pleasurable experience for the mother, elective C-section is far more dangerous to mother and child. Recovery is slower after C-section and breastfeeding is more often unsuccessful. Multiple drugs are used for Cesarean surgery, and those drugs enter the baby's circulation. In addition, the skin-to-skin mother-infant bonding period that occurs just after a vaginal birth is impossible after a C-section.

Breastfeeding and Probiotics

Breast milk contains living probiotics. Breast-fed babies receive repeated doses of living probiotics; babies fed on formula do not. Again, this could at least partially explain the link between formula feeding and gastrointestinal problems—problems likely compounded by the fact that cow's milk can be allergenic, especially to the immature GI tract of an infant. Researchers have isolated an antibacterial carbohydrate called *reuterin* from breast milk; this carbohydrate likely helps to prevent infection in infants' GI tracts.

Formula manufacturers are catching on to the need for probiotics in infants, and are making products that contain *Lactobacillus rhamnosus*; this is a step in the right direction, but doesn't match the natural growth of bacteria specific to infants that occurs with breastfeeding. The primary forms of probiotic that first colonize a baby's GI tract are *Bifidobacteria*, with lesser amounts of *L. rhamnosus*, *L. paracasei*, and *L. salivarius*.

During the first days of nursing, the mother's breasts make a watery food known as colostrum. Colostrum doesn't have much in the way of calories, but it's loaded with antibodies. These antibodies establish the baby's intestinal immune system and immunity throughout his or her body. Colostrum also contains growth factors that help the GI tract to ready itself for mother's milk. Without colostrum, immunity is bound to suffer. Parents of any infant who is not going to be breast-fed would do well to consider giving the infant bovine (from cows) colostrum with the guidance of a pediatrician.

The development of gut immunity is also hampered when a baby is exclusively formula-fed, and every feeding at the mother's breast enhances the formation of this important aspect of the immune system. Fecal analysis of formula-fed babies shows that pathogenic *enterococci*, *coliform*, and *clostridia* dominate the gastrointestinal ecosystem; the flora of breast-fed infants, on the other hand, are made up primarily of beneficial *staphylococci* and bifidobacteria. In breast-fed infants, bifidobacteria are also the predominant fecal flora until weaning.

It follows that every mother who is able to do so should breastfeed for as long as possible. Although nursing past the first six months is practically unheard of in the United States, the World Health Organization recommends nursing for at least a year (with, of course, the introduction of solid foods after six months). Some mothers choose to nurse for two or more years, and this helps to ease the transition into a healthful solid food diet. Mothers who can't nurse should consider supplementing baby's formula with a powdered probiotic supplement made especially for this purpose, with the guidance of the baby's pediatrician.

Infant and Childhood Diarrhea Controlled with Probiotics

In undeveloped nations, more than 600,000 children die from rotavirus diarrhea each year. The use of probiotics as a diarrhea preventative and treatment could be of huge help in these nations. Probiotic supplementation has been found to decrease the shedding of rotavirus—an indication that probiotics have antiviral activity that shortens the duration and decreases contagion of this disease. In two reviews of studies on acute infectious diarrhea in infants and children, it was found that probiotic therapy decreased the duration of acute diarrhea by twenty to just under twenty-nine hours. One group of researchers supplemented the formula of hospitalized infants with *Streptococcus thermophilus,* a friendly bacteria. Over a period of seventeen months, 31 percent of infants not given the probiotic supplement developed diarrhea, in comparison to only seven percent of probiotic-fed babies.

Twenty to 40 percent of the children who are prescribed broad-spectrum antibiotics each year end up with diarrhea as a result; with 30.3 million antibiotic prescriptions written for United States' children each year, this is not an insignificant problem. Researchers at the University of Nebraska evaluated the effects of 10 billion colony forming units (CFU) of *L. casei* on antibiotic-associated diarrhea in children. They found that *L. casei* decreased the incidence of diarrhea by 75 percent after ten days.

One in every 800 children suffers from Crohn's disease, an inflammatory illness that causes GI pain, cramping, and recurrent diarrhea. Probiotics are an important aspect of Crohn's disease therapy; they decrease inflammation and help to normalize gut immunity. Interestingly, the work of autism researcher Andrew Wakefield has shown a link between Crohn's-like gut problems and autism. This may be why a non-allergenic diet has proven helpful in autistic children in a study by Athos Bousvaros at Children's Hospital in Boston, Mass.

Certain strains of *Lactobacillus* have been shown to promote recovery from rotavirus enteritis in hospitalized children. In a study published in *The Pediatric Infectious Disease Journal,* researchers found that in children from day-care centers with mild gastroenteritis, combination strains of *Lactobacilli* were effective in reducing the duration of diarrhea.

Infant Candidiasis and Probiotics

An overgrowth of *candida* can cause either oral thrush or a severe form of diaper rash (also known as *candida diaper dermatitis*). Oral thrush is a common condition in nursing babies. Older children who use steroid inhalers for asthma may also develop oral thrush.

The appearance of oral thrush in infants can be tricky to decipher; it's easy to mistake the natural whitish coating created by frequent intake of rich breast milk for candida. A baby with thrush will have a white film or patches on the tongue, the inner surfaces of the cheeks, or on the roof of the mouth. While milk coating these parts of the mouth can be easily scraped off with a cotton swab, candida can't be removed this way.

Generally, thrush causes no discomfort to the baby. It can, however, be transferred to the mother's nipple, and this can cause her to develop an itchy, burning rash that makes nursing difficult. Mainstream treatment usually involves an antifungal drug such as nystatin, which must be prescribed by a physician. Probiotics are a better bet; they'll correct the bacterial imbalance that causes the overgrowth in the first place. Swab the baby's mouth with a cotton swab dipped in a solution of baby probiotic powder and water or breast milk once a day. Sprinkle a small amount of the same powder on mom's nipples if they are affected by the yeast. The nursing mother with thrush on her nipple should also take a probiotic supplement daily, and follow the guidelines for an anti-yeast diet as described in Chapter 2. Also be sure to change nursing pads with each feeding and boil any bottle nipples or pacifiers following each use.

Candida diaper dermatitis is intensely red. Small red extensions may be seen along the edges of the rash. Topical antifungal medications may be necessary to treat severe diaper rash; try a baby probiotic supplement, as well. Other basic measures for controlling diaper rash include promptly changing soiled diapers (prolonged exposure to urine or feces is a major cause of diaper rash) and letting baby's bottom air-dry after cleaning.

Probiotics Are Useful for More Serious Pediatric Health Problems

Generally, the digestive systems of children born with HIV infection are a mess. They have chronic episodes of diarrhea, tend toward pathogenic bacterial overgrowth, and have trouble absorbing adequate nutrients from the foods they eat. In one study of seventeen children with HIV, some received *L. plantarum* 299v and others received a placebo. The probiotic improved the childrens' height and weight more than the placebo, and many of the children had small improvements in immune response; one subject's immune function was almost completely normalized after the probiotic therapy. There were no adverse effects in any of the children who took probiotics.

In rare instances, newborns will develop *neonatal necrotizing entero-colitis* (NEC), a potentially fatal digestive disorder. Researchers developed a laboratory model of NEC and found that the probiotic *Bifidobacterium infantis* significantly reduced the likelihood of its development.

If you are interested in giving beneficial bacteria to an infant or a child under the age of two, please make sure you use a form specially made for babies. Older children can use a wider range of bacteria—those found in probiotic supplements for adults—without problems.

CHAPTER 8

OTHER BENEFITS
OF PROBIOTICS

Just in case you aren't yet convinced that you are better off using pro-biotic supplements than not, here are some accounts of promising research into even more uses for these amazing microorganisms!

Cholesterol Lowering

The Masai people have long been a thorn in the side of the theory that high-meat, high-fat, high-cholesterol diets are the reason why heart attacks happen. These African cattle-herding people eat mostly milk and meat, and their cholesterol levels are low and heart disease is virtually unheard of in their tribes. The most up-to-date research is showing that excess sugar and refined carbohydrates may be more of a problem than milk and meat, which are, after all, natural, whole foods. But there may be another reason why the Masai thrive on their high-cholesterol fare: they use probiotic bacteria to ferment much of the milk they consume.

Bacterial populations in the intestinal tract strongly influence the syn-thesis, absorption, and metabolism of cholesterol. Several studies have shown that *L. acidophilus* (DDS-1) takes up cholesterol in lab-created environments identical to those in the intestinal tract. Studies on both animals and humans have shown that fermented milk—otherwise known as yogurt—contains an *anticholesterolemic milk factor* (AMF) that appears to inhibit the activity of a liver enzyme needed for cholesterol synthesis. The regular consumption of yogurt and acidophilus milk has been found to have cholesterol-lowering effects.

In one study, researchers fed rats with regular milk, which didn't cause their cholesterol to rise. They then added cholesterol to their diets and their blood cholesterol rose as a result. Adding 4 million *L. acidophilus* DDS-1 per milliliter of milk brought cholesterol levels down significantly.

Liver Health

The liver is the body's most important cleansing organ. When its function suffers—often due to the use of prescription drugs, or to overconsumption of alcohol—toxins build up in the body. One toxic chemical that accumulates during liver failure is ammonia. If not remedied, this buildup can cause brain swelling, disturbances in consciousness, tremors, coma, and even death. Probiotics have ammonia-lowering effects.

People with liver cirrhosis have imbalanced microflora. Antibiotics are often given to cirrhosis patients to reduce the production of bacterial toxins that contribute to increased blood pressure in the portal vein, which feeds the liver. It has been hypothesized that probiotics could have the same effect on this liver-damaging portal hypertension.

Harvard researchers found that these bacterial good guys improved mental function and overall clinical status in patients with liver failure. At the New England Deaconess Hospital in Boston, Massachusetts, researchers showed that *L. acidophilus* fed to lab animals reduced the risk of endotoxemia and the severity of damage due to experimental alcoholic liver disease.

In a study on human alcohol cirrhosis patients, researchers found that several months' worth of treatment with *B. bifidum* and *L. acidophilus* improved ammonia levels and improved mental status and psychological performance better than patients who were given diuretics and lactulose. Of the patients that were hospitalized, the probiotic-treated ones went home sooner than those who were given drugs.

Kidney Health

The kidneys are also important cleansing organs; kidney failure causes toxins to accumulate in the blood, and dialysis doesn't do much to reduce their levels. Japanese researchers have shown that probiotics reduce the workload on the kidneys by decreasing the production of bacterial toxins in the body.

Aging

People over the age of fifty are more prone to gastrointestinal complaints. This is due, in part, to a natural age-related decrease in populations of beneficial microflora relative to pathogenic bugs like *clostridia* and *enterococci*. Supplementing with probiotics and helping their populations along with the right foods is a good idea for anyone wanting to grow old gracefully, and with a minimum of gastrointestinal distress!

Probiotics for Pets

If you're ever in the mood to read publications for those who raise livestock, you'll find that the probiotic revolution is already happening in barnyards across the nation. With the prevalence of antibiotic resistance, farmers are finally seeing the wisdom of using natural remedies, including probiotics, to enhance their animals' health and growth. Plenty of research supports the use of probiotics for this purpose.

The animals with which we share our homes and our love are increasingly fed on processed foods. This has the same effect on their flora that human processed diets have on human flora, and gastrointestinal problems can often result. Animals on processed diets are also more vulnerable to cancer, allergies, and arthritis—all problems that have been widely helped with probiotic supplements.

Check with your vet or pet store to find out whether they have begun to carry probiotics tailored to your furry (or feathery) friends, or seek some out on the Internet.

Probiotics for Large Animals

In the 1950s, probiotics were used as a drug to combat *E. coli* infection in pigs. Today, probiotics are used by farmers for all large animals and chickens for growth promotion, for production, and as an antibacterial agent.

CHAPTER 9

CHOOSING AND USING PROBIOTIC SUPPLEMENTS

With more than 400 strains of beneficial microorganisms to choose from, you might fear that the search for the best possible probiotic will be a difficult one. Quality control is another problematic issue when it comes to probiotics, which aren't effective unless they get into your body while alive and kicking. A recent test run by independent laboratory ConsumerLab. com found that many probiotic supplements had only one percent of the billion-plus organisms you need. Some had only a ten-thousandth of a percent. All in all, a quarter of the probiotics analyzed didn't meet the expectations laid out on their labels.

The major categories of probiotic bacteria are lactobacilli and bifidobacteria. Strains of these two bacteria have been thoroughly studied for both safety and effectiveness. These strains are used in the making of yogurt and other fermented foods, and are packaged in the form of supplements.

Including Probiotics in Your Diet

Promoting healthy microflora balance isn't only about taking a supplement. Beneficial microorganisms can be cultivated with the right foods, as well. No supplement is going to fix the problem of a poor diet.

Yogurt is the best known fermented food. Yogurt cultures are often not those specifically found in the GI tract, but they still have beneficial effects and are able to colonize the intestinal tract and bring you all of the benefits that have been discussed in this book. Even lactose-intolerant people can usually tolerate yogurt, because the good bugs pre-digest the lactose it contains. Choose a brand that's organic, preferably plain; the flavored varieties tend to contain a lot of sugar. Make sure the yogurt you buy contains live cultures that were added *after* pasteurization (pasteurization kills all bacteria) and enjoy a little each day.

Please note that probiotic bacteria do not last long in yogurt. Watch for the viability of probiotic bacteria.

Not sure you're crazy about plain yogurt? It might seem a bit sour at first compared to flavored varieties. Luckily, there are lots of healthful ways to jazz it up. Try:

- Adding fresh fruit.
- Adding organic granola.
- Dolloping yogurt onto a steaming bowl of oatmeal.
- Using it instead of sour cream.
- Adding a tiny bit of maple syrup.
- Adding a tablespoon of flaxseed meal or wheat germ.
- Using it as a base for salad dressings and dips.

As you enjoy your yogurt, keep in mind that the addition of probiotic cultures to milk increases the bioavailability of calcium, iron, magnesium, potassium, phosphorus, zinc, and most of the B vitamins. Yogurt cheese is a good alternative to cream cheese. More adventuresome readers might be interested in making their own yogurt, or cheeses made from yogurt; check the Resources section for books on how to do so.

If you aren't a yogurt fan, try one of the available brands of acidophilus milk. You should be able to find it in your local health food store. Kefir is widely sold, but it tends to be loaded with sugar. Those who choose to avoid milk completely can get probiotics from fermented soy products, including soy yogurt and tempeh (an Asian food that can be used in stir-fries or chili, or can be made into a vegetarian sloppy Joe).

Take It Easy on the Meat

Small portions of lean meat are part of a well-rounded whole-foods diet. Too much meat, however, encourages the growth of putrefactive bacteria, which in turn increases colon cancer risk.

A serving of meat, fish, or chicken should be the size of a deck of playing cards, and you need not have these foods at every meal. Try getting some of your protein from nuts, beans, or tofu rather than relying completely on flesh foods. And, of course, buy free-range or organic meats whenever possible. They taste better and are better for the environment, and they aren't dosed up on the antibiotics given to conventional livestock.

The Importance of Prebiotics

Yes, you read it right: not probiotics, but *prebiotics*. Prebiotics are the preferred foods of the beneficial bugs that live in your colon. The probiotics are also nourished by the contents of your intestines, and they are fairly choosy about what they'll consume. Supplying probiotics with the foods they like enables them to produce the nutrients, short-chain fatty acids, amino acids, growth factors, antioxidants, and vitamins required by the cells that line your colon.

Prebiotics are elements of the foods we eat that can't be broken down by enzymes in the small intestine. This is one way in which a whole-foods diet rich in fiber supports the health of the GI tract. Typical low-fiber processed-food diets, on the other hand, don't give colon flora the fuel they require to do their jobs, although they supply plenty of fuel for *Candida* yeast.

The favored food of colon bacteria are a group of complex carbohydrates called *oligosaccharides*. These carbohydrates resist being broken down by the salivary and small intestinal enzymes that break down virtually every other component of the foods we eat. Once they reach the colon, they are fermented by the bacteria that reside there.

Fructooligosaccharides (FOS)—a type of oligosaccharide—selectively stimulate the growth of probiotics. This, in turn, reduces the population of pathogenic bacteria. FOS occurs naturally in vegetables and fruits such as bananas, garlic, wheat, onion, tomato, and barley. Inulin is another prebiotic often added to probiotic supplements.

Prebiotics selectively feed probiotics, not pathogenic bacteria. It is also indigestible by us.

Current dietary guidelines suggest that 20 percent of total food consumed be comprised of oligosaccharides. This means a diet that contains lots of fiber-rich whole foods—fruits, vegetables, beans, and whole grains.

The best probiotic supplements must contain prebiotics. Combinations of pro- and prebiotics have been termed "symbiotics."

How to Choose a Good Probiotic Supplement

Any probiotic found in a supplement has been tested to ensure that it's safe, but some are better than others at promoting optimal health. To qualify as a beneficial microorganism, a bacterium must meet the following criteria:

- Be acid- and bile-resistant so that it can make the journey to the intestines without being destroyed by acid or bile.
- Reduce the pH of the colon.
- Be metabolically active in the GI tract.
- Possess antimicrobial activity against pathogenic bacteria.
- Demonstrate the ability to adhere to and colonize the GI tract.
- Modulate immunity in a positive way.
- Demonstrate the ability to reduce intestinal permeability.
- Must be safe to the human body—generally recognized as safe (GRAS).

Ideally, the probiotic supplement you choose should contain *L. acidophilus* and/or other *Lactobacillus* strains and strains of *Bifidobacterium* fortified with FOS (prebiotics). Here's a list of specific probiotic strains you might find in supplements:

Bifidobacterium longum

Bifidobacterium infantis

Bifidobacterium bifidum

Lactobacillus acidophilus

Lactobacillus casei

Lactobacillus lactis

Lactobacillus plantarum

Lactobacillus reuteri

Lactobacillus rhamnosus

Lactobacillus salivarius

Streptococcus thermophilus

No supplement usually contains all of these bacteria.

Probiotic supplement activity is measured in CFU, or colony forming units. A healthy person's daily dose should contain 2 to 5 billion CFU. Those with gastrointestinal problems can take up to 10 billion CFU a day.

Probiotics are safe even in doses far greater than anyone would intentionally take. In extremely rare instances, seriously ill people have developed infections caused by supposedly "good" bacteria. If you have severe immune dysfunction or some other kind of life-threatening illness, check with your doctor before trying probiotics.

What Form to Use

Available forms include capsules, tablets, powders, and liquids. Most people prefer the ease of capsules or tablets. Powders should be mixed with unchilled water and taken ten to thirty minutes before a meal. Liquids tend to be unstable and aren't generally recommended by probiotics experts. Children can take powdered forms mixed with juice or milk. Powders or capsules that can be opened to pour the powder out are best for rinsing the mouth or using to treat yeast infections on the breast or in the vagina.

Although some strains may not require refrigeration, it's always best to keep them refrigerated. Most strains are stable at temperatures under 40°F. Don't leave probiotics in a hot car or in a sunny spot. Protect your probiotic supplements from heat, moisture, and oxygen. The best brands are packaged in amber glass bottles to decrease the contact of light with the bacteria.

Choose a brand that carries an expiration date on the bottle. It should indicate that the bacteria were tested for viability upon packaging. If you have concerns or questions about the probiotic supplement you've chosen, contact the manufacturer and ask them whether it meets the standards listed in this chapter.

CHAPTER 10

NEW RESEARCH
INTO PROBIOTIC BENEFITS

The benefits of probiotics are numerous, and ongoing research seems to reveal more and more benefits with every passing day. One of the most exciting recent developments is in diabetic men and women, where daily consumption of probiotics has been shown to reduce fat, blood pressure, and blood glucose. A second field of study that will undoubtedly become a hot topic in the coming years is that of psychobiotics, which are bacteria that reside in your intestines and improve your mental health.

Additional new developments will also be seen in the following areas:

- **Prebiotics**—Whole food ingredients that nurture the probiotics *and* your own gut bacteria.

- **Combined probiotics**—The concept of cultivating diverse probiotic strains together, resulting in a synergistic effect.

- **Postbiotics**—Organic acids, chelated minerals (those that have been chemically combined with amino acids to form complexes), enzymes, and other health-promoting nutrients created by live, active probiotics.

Benefits of Probiotics

Hundreds of pages could be written—and, in fact, *have* been written—about the varied benefits of taking probiotics. A few examples are:

- When given to participants for one month, *Lactobacillus helveticus* (the bacterium used in the production of American Swiss Cheese) and

Bifidobacterium longum showed markedly decreased cortisol levels, resulting in better moods for the participants.

- Certain probiotics have been shown to regulate the action of pro-inflammatory cytokines, too many of which have been linked to memory loss, depression, and cognitive and mood disorders.
- *Hu36 Bacillus indicus* strains produce RDA levels of calcium in your intestines, where they are immediately absorbed.

Reducing Kids' Need for Antibiotics

It is common and alarming knowledge that the levels of antibiotic resistance (2 million cases and 23,000 deaths each year in the United States) is growing. Fortunately, it has been shown that giving daily probiotic supplements to children can reduce their likelihood of even needing antibiotics.

A study in the *European Journal of Public Health* showed that infants and children who took daily probiotic supplements were 29 percent less likely to have been prescribed antibiotics. The study considered twelve different studies; the rate was increased to 53 percent when the highest quality studies were factored.

Senior investigator Daniel Merenstein, MD, says: "We don't know all the mechanisms probiotic strains may leverage, but since most of the human immune system is found in the gastrointestinal tract, ingesting healthy bacteria may competitively exclude bacterial pathogens linked to gut infections and may prime the immune system to fight others."

Gut Microbiome Alterations in Alzheimer's Disease

It is estimated that nearly 6 million people over the age of 65—nearly one in 10—have Alzheimer's disease. A recent study revealed that "the gut microbiome (the microorganisms in a particular environment) of Alzheimer's disease participants has decreased microbial diversity."

Although the research is ongoing, seeing a change to the microbiomes of Alzheimer's patients is potentially important. After all, our bodies depend on a vast army of microbiomes to stay alive; they protect us against germs, break down food to release energy, and produce vitamins.

The Latest Developments

New and hopeful studies on the benefits of probiotics seem to be published every day. Some of the more exciting recent developments are:

- Probiotics have been shown to improve gut symptoms (such as irritable bowel syndrome) and lessen anxiety. In a study of patients with irritable bowel syndrome, 69 percent of those who took a multistrain probiotic reported a decrease in abdominal pain, compared to 47 percent who took a placebo.

- Georgia-based Deerland Enzymes & Probiotics announced that its proprietary branded probiotic strain *Bacillus subtilis* DE111 was granted non-Novel Food ingredient status in Canada. *B. subtilis* DE111 differs from most probiotic strains in its ability to produce protective spores. This company has also produced a more soluble form of its probiotic strain DE111.

- A Canadian-based company, Lallemand Health Solutions, has been granted the right to claim that its *Lactobacillus helveticus* LAFTI L10 strain "promotes gastrointestinal health in physically active adults."

100 Million Neurons Strong

People are often shocked—perhaps even horrified—when they learn that the bacteria in their gut weighs up to three or four pounds. Equally as interesting is the fact that your intestines contain **100 million** neurons which allow you to "feel" the inside of your body. Some people even refer to this as "the second brain." Certain types of bacteria can hook up to this "second brain" and affect how you think, feel, and react to stress.

The population of probiotics in every person's gut is unique, not unlike a person's fingerprints. Of the trillions of individuals of probiotics, belonging to thousands of known species, it is estimated that 85 percent of probiotics are beneficial, while 15 percent are detrimental. The good probiotics assist with digestion and breaking down toxins. Furthermore, they help to prevent a myriad of conditions such as obesity, diabetes, neurodegenerative disorders, and heart disease.

Psychobiotics

Psychobiotics are, for the most part, normal probiotics, although they perform roles other than those performed by "normal" gut bacteria. Many health professionals view psychobiotics as "the new frontier in the treatment of mental illnesses like depression and anxiety."

One study showed that giving mice the probiotic *Lactobacillus rhamnosus* significantly reduced their levels of stress, anxiety, and depression.

Notably, the same effect did *not* occur in mice whose vagus nerve (the cranial nerve that facilitates communication between the brain and the intestines) was severed.

When discussing the benefits of probiotics, much of the discussion naturally centers on a person's gut—after all, the microbes that reside in your gut help to synthesize neurotransmitters (chemicals the brain cells use to relay messages to and from each other) such as serotonin, gaba, dopamine, acetylcholine, and norepinephrine. This is not insignificant, as over 90 percent of the serotonin and 50 percent of the dopamine in your body is found in your gut.

Other promising uses of psychobiotics are:

- They can help to lessen brain inflammation, which can cause depression.

- They can promote the formation of new brain cells, which helps in preventing Huntington's disease and Alzheimer's disease.

- The can help protect your brain from damage—specifically, psychobiotics can help prevent oxidative damage brought about by the action of oxygen-carrying free radicals.

The Popularity of Probiotics

It has been estimated that more than 60 million people in the United States are dealing with some sort of gut issue. It has also been estimated that the cost of treating these ailments is approximately $100 billion per year. Moreover, more than 100 million visits are made to physicians each year related to digestive issues.

If probiotics can aid in these digestive issues, their increased prevalence could have an overall positive effect on our society.

In the "olden days," probiotics were "relegated to the refrigerators of health food stores," and the people who took them were rabid health-food junkies who rushed their probiotics home to stick in their own refrigerators.

That was then, and this is now. According to the *Nutrition Business Journal*, gastrointestinal health makes up nearly 7 percent (or $1.9 billion) of the U.S. supplement market—a number that is expected to rise in the coming years.

The increasing popularity—and acceptance—of probiotics can be attributed to several factor such as:

- Increased media exposure.

- The increased number of medical practitioners recommending probiotics to their patients.
- Increasing knowledge of the consumer.

Sheryl Eaglewoman, a manager of Mountain Valley Foods in Montana, says: "Consumers seem to know (more about) the relationship between the gut and other organs such as the brain and heart. They are also more knowledgeable about the critical role of prebiotics."
The increased popularity of probiotics has resulted in some exciting new milestones, such as:

- The ability to freeze/spray dry the product, which prolongs the life of many probiotics in supplements.
- The introduction of spore-based probiotics, which increasingly survive digestion (it is estimated that 10 to 30 percent of probiotics survive going down the gastrointestinal tract).
- The single-dose probiotic (SingleDaily Probiotics), which is offered in 10 billion, 30 billion, and 50 billion CFU (colony-forming unit) strengths. These have been tailored to target such specific areas as colon and vaginal health.

Raw Probiotics

There are dozens of reasons why somebody might choose to take a probiotic—and many people take these in the forms of daily probiotic supplements. According to Bruce Topping, a probiotic expert: "If you do (take a daily probiotic supplement), then you should look for a raw, whole food probiotic supplement that is designed for your exact needs."

Why does Topping suggest that your probiotic be raw? Well, in his words: "To be blunt—heat kills." In other words, if you are ingesting bacteria that is supposed to be beneficial to your gut, it needs to be alive when it reaches your gut. He therefore recommends finding a probiotic that is "carefully manufactured in a climate- and humidity-controlled environment, stored in a cool warehouse, and shipped cold and kept in the store's cooler rather than on the store's shelf."

Probiotics and Plants

If probiotic products are good for human health, it seems logical that the plants we grow might also benefit from certain microbes—which should theoretically benefit the environment as a whole.

In an article in the *American Society of Agronomy*, Kaine Korzewka describes how legumes (beans, peas, lentils) have beneficial bacteria in nodules attached to their roots; these bacteria turn nitrogen into a form the plant can use. Korzewka explains how, "researchers have recently found some nitrogen-fixing bacteria actually live inside plant tissue—in the leaves, stems, and roots—with impressive results."

How does this benefit the environment as a whole? According to Korzewka: "Thanks to these bacteria fixing nitrogen for the plant, farmers could use less chemical fertilizers to give plants the nitrogen they need." Using less fertilizer benefits the surrounding ecosystems and even decreases greenhouse gas emissions.

Probiotics in Food and Agricultural Science

Probiotics can be found in several commercial dairy products such as sour and fresh milk, yogurt, and cheese. These products "play an important role in delivering probiotic bacteria to humans, as these products provide a suitable environment for probiotic bacteria that support their growth and viability."

This is good news for people who consume dairy—but did you know that an astonishing 65 percent of the world's population is lactose intolerant? Fortunately, fermented vegetables are another way in which humans can ingest probiotics. Some examples of the many potential non-dairy foods are:

• Vegetable-based drinks

• Peanut milk

• Cranberry, pineapple, and orange juices

• Fermented soymilk drinks

• Rice-based yogurt

• Maize-based beverages

In addition to these products, there is much research being done throughout the world in fruit-based, cereal-based, and meat-based probiotic products. Furthermore, scientists are, to cite two examples, examining the benefits of adding probiotics to chicken and pig feed, which will help with the health of consumable animals.

CONCLUSION

The evidence in support of probiotics for optimal health is over-whelming. Even mainstream medicine is being forced to take notice. Using friendly natural microorganisms to combat less friendly varieties runs counter to the medical mainstream's usual "magic bullet" techniques for dealing with disease, but there's no denying that it works. Probiotic therapy is also cheaper and far more safe than antibiotics and the drugs used to counter the inflammatory diseases and yeast problems that can result from intestinal bacterial imbalances.

Many probiotics researchers have expressed hope that the intelligent use of probiotics could be the answer to the frightening problem of antibiotic resistance. If this problem is not dealt with, antibiotics—which are, to be fair, as close to a "miracle drug" as any ever developed—will be rendered useless. Providing the body with better natural defenses against pathogenic bacteria will allow doctors to only use antibiotics when absolutely necessary.

Probiotics are being employed in the treatment and prevention of bad breath, ulcers, indigestion, leaky gut, food allergy, inflammatory bowel disease, constipation, diarrhea, irritable bowel syndrome, sys-temic and local yeast infections, acne, eczema, and rheumatoid arthritis. They show promise for the prevention of cancer, particularly those that strike the gastrointestinal tract. The health of infants and children can also be dramatically improved with appropriate use of probiotics.

These beneficial bugs deserve a place right alongside a high-quality multivitamin and mineral supplement as an essential part of your daily nutrition plan.

It is wise to use a good quality probiotic supplement containing *Lactobacillus* and *Bifidus,* and fortified with FOS, on a daily basis to maintain good healthy flora to defend against infection.

SELECTED REFERENCES

Adak A, Khan MR. An insight into gut microbiota and its functionalities. Cell Mol Life Sci. 2018 Oct 13. [PubMed 30317530]

Alm L. "Acidophilus milk for therapy in gastrointestinal disorders." *Nahrung*, 1984;28(6–7):683–4.

Anderson JW and Gilliland SE. "Effect of fermented milk (yogurt) containing Lactobacillus acidophilus L1 on serum cholesterol in hypercholesterolemic humans." *J Am Coll Nutr*, 1999 Feb;18(1):43–50.

Bagchi D and Dash SK. "*Lactobacillus acidophilus:* Natural Antibiotics and Beyond." *Townsend Letter for Doctors and Patients*, 1996 Feb/Mar.

Bengmark S. "Colonic food: pre- and probiotics." *Am J Gastroenterol*, 2000;95(Suppl):S5-S7.

Biffi A, et al. "Antiproliferative effect of fermented milk on the growth of a human breast cancer cell line." *Nutr Cancer*, 1997;28(1):93–9.

Borglund E, Hagermark O, Nord CE. "Impact of topical clindamycin and systemic tetracycline on the skin and colon microflora in patients with acne vulgaris." *Scand J Infect Dis Suppl*, 1984;43:76–81.

Brashears MM, Gilliland SE, Buck LM. "Bile salt deconjugation and cholesterol removal from media by Lactobacillus casei." *J Dairy Sci*, 1998 Aug;81(8): 2103–10.

Buck L, et al. "Comparisons of freshly isolated strains of L. acidophilus of human intestinal origin for ability to assimilate cholesterol during growth." *J Dairy Sci*, 1994;77:2925–33.

Caplan MS and Jilling T. "Neonatal necrotizing enterocolitis: possible role of probiotic supplements." *J Pediatr Gastroenterol Nutr*, 2000; 3 Suppl 2:S18–22.

Chaitow L and Natasha Trenev. 1990. *Probiotics*. Wellingboro, England: Thorsons Publishing Group.

Coconnier MH, et al. "Antagonistic activity against Helicobacter pylori infection in vitro and in vivo by human Lactobacillus acidophilus strain LB." *Appl Environ Microbiol*, 1998 Nov;64(11):4573–80.

Colle R and Ceschia T. "Oral bacteriotherapy with bifidobacterium bifidum and lactobacillus acidophilus in cirrhotic patients." *Clin Ter*, 1989 Dec 31;131(6): 397–402.

Cremon C, Barbaro Mr, Ventura M, Barbara G. Pre- and probiotic overview. Curr Opin Pharmacol. 2018 Sep 13; 43; 87-92. [PubMed 30219638]

Crook, William G, Hyla Cass, and Elizabeth B Crook. *The Yeast Connection and Women's Health*. Professional Books, February 2003.

Cunningham-Rundles S, et al. "Probiotics and immune response." *Am J Gastroenterol*, 2000;95: S22–25.

Dash SK. "How to select an Acidophilus supplement." *The Garden Within*, 1989;12–18.

Dash SK, Spreen Alan N, and Ley Beth M. "Health Benefits of Probiotics." BL Publications, 2002.

Dash SK. "The Surprising Story Behind Probiotics." *The Doctor's Prescription for Healthy Living*, 2002; 6 (11).

Delia P, et al. "Prevention of radiation-induced diarrhea with the use of VSL#3, a new high-potency probiotic preparation." *Am J Gastroenterol*, 2002 Aug; 97(8):2150–2.

deRoos NM, Katan MB. "Effects of probiotic bacteria on diarrhea, lipid metabolism, and carcinogenesis: a review of papers published between 1988 and 1998." *Am J Clin Nutr*, 2000 Feb;71(2):405–11.

Drisko JA, Giles CK, Bischoff RD. "Probiotics in Health Maintenance and Disease Prevention." *Alternative Medicine Review*, 2003;8(2):143–55.

Foltz-Gray, Dorothy. "Why You Should Eat Bugs." *Alternative Medicine*, 2003 June:42.

Friedlander A, Tomioka H, Ohkido S. "Lactobacillus acidophilus and vitamin B complex in the treatment of vaginal infection." *Panminerva Med*, 1986;28: 51–53.

Frutos MJ, Valero-Cases E, Rincon-Frutos L. Food components with potential to be used in the therapeutic approach of mental diseases. Curr Pharm Biotechnol. 2018 Sep 25. [PubMed 30346890]

Fuller R. "Probiotics in human medicine." *Gut*, 1991; 32:439–42.

Gronlund MM, et al. "Mode of delivery directs the phagocyte functions of infants for the first 6 months of life." *Clin Exp Immunol*, 1999 Jun;116(3):521–6.

Health Canada Grants *Lactobacillus helveticus* LAFTI L10 New Health Claims

Hida M, et al. "Inhibition of the accumulation of uremic toxins in the blood and their precursors in the feces after oral administration of Lebenin, a lactic acid bacteria preparation, to uremic patients undergoing hemodialysis." *Nephron*, 1996;74(2): 349–55.

Hilton E, et al. "Ingested yoghurt as prophylaxis for chronic candidal vaginitis." *Ann Intern Med*, 1992; 116:353–7.

Isolauri F, Kirjavainen PV, Salminen S. "Probiotics: a role in the treatment of intestinal infection and inflammation?" *Gut*, 2002 May;50 Suppl 3:III54–9.

Jhonson, RJ. "Psychobiotics: Intestinal bacteria that improve your mental health." *Natural News*. August 5, 2018.

Kalliomaki M and Isolauri E. "Role of intestinal flora in the development of allergy." *Curr Opin Allergy Clin Immunol*, 2003 Feb;3(1):15–20.

Kalliomaki M, et al. "Probiotics in primary prevention of atopic disease: a randomised placebo-controlled trial." *Lancet*, 2003 May 31;361(9372):1869–71.

Kirjavainen PV, et al. "Aberrant composition of gut microbiota of allergic infants: a target of bifidobacterial therapy at weaning?" *Gut*, 2002 Jul;51(1):51–5.

Kirjavainen PV, et al. "The effect of orally administered viable probiotic and dairy lactobacilli on mouse lymphocyte proliferation." *FEMS Immunol Med Microbiol*, 1999 Nov;26(2):131–5.

Kontiokari T, et al. "Dietary factors protecting women from urinary tract infection." *Am J Clin Nutr*, 2003 Mar;77(3):600–4.

Korzewka, Kaine. "Probiotics—for Plants." *American Society of Agronomy*. July 8, 2015. https://agronomy.org/science-news/probiotics-plants

Kuo PH, Chung YE. Moody microbiome: Challenges and chances. J Formos Med Assoc. 2018 Sep 25. [PubMed 30262220]

Landau, Kara, APD/AN. "Prebiotics: The New Gut Health Nutrient Driving Product Innovation." *Insider*. November/December 2018: 116.

Lappe, Marc. 1997. *The Tao of Immunology*. New York, NY: Plenum Trade Publishing.

Levy A, Conway JM, Dangl JL, Woyke T. Elucidating Bacterial Gene Functions in the Plant Microbiome. Cell Host Microbe. 2018 Oct 10; 24(4): 475-485. [PubMed 30308154]

Liu Y, Alookaran JJ, Rhoads JM. Probiotics in Autoimmune and Inflammatory Disorders. Nutrients. 2018 Oct 18: 10(10). [PubMed 30340338]

Mack DR, et al. "Probiotics inhibit enteropathogenic E. coli adherence in vitro by inducing intestinal mucin gene expression." *Am J Physiol*, 1999;276:G941– G950.

Madsen KL, et al. "Normal breast milk limits the development of colitis in IL-10 deficient mice." *Inflamm Bowel Dis*, 2002 Nov;8(6):390–8.

Majamaa H, Isolauri E. "Probiotics: a novel approach in the management of food allergy." *J Allergy Clin Immunol*, 1997;99:179–85.

Malin M, et al. "Dietary therapy with Lactobacillus GG, bovine colostrums or bovine immune colostrums in patients with juvenile chronic arthritis: evaluation of effect of gut defense mechanisms." *Inflammopharmacology*, 1997;5:219–236.

Marchetti F, et al. "Efficacy of regulators of the intestinal bacterial flora in the therapy of acne vulgaris." *Clin Ter*, 1987 Sep 15;122(5):339–43.

Marotta, Ryan. "Daily Probiotics May Reduce Kids' Needs for Antibiotics." September 14, 2018. https://www.pharmacytimes.com/resource-centers/vitamins-supplements

Marteau PR. "Probiotics in clinical conditions." *Clin Rev Allergy Immunol*, 2002 Jun;22(3):255–73.

Midolo PD, et al. "In vitro inhibition of Helicobacter pylori NCTC 11637 by organic acids and lactic acid bacteria." *J Appl Bacteriol*, 1995;79:475–79.

Miraglia del Giudice M Jr, De Luca MG, Capristo C. "Probiotics and atopic dermatitis. A new strategy in atopic dermatitis." *Dig Liver Dis*, 2002 Sep; 34 Suppl 2:S68–71.

Murch SH. "Toll of allergy reduced by probiotics." *Lancet*, 2001;357:1057–1059.

Nanji AA, Khettry U, Sadrzadeh SM. "Lactobacillus feeding reduces endotoxemia and severity of experimental alcoholic liver disease." *Proc Soc Exp Biol Med*, 1994 Mar;205(3):243–7.

Niedzielin K, Kordecki H, Birkenfeld B. "A controlled, double-blind, randomized study on the efficacy of Lactobacillus plantarum 299V in patients with irritable bowel syndrome." *Eur J Gastroenterol Hepatol*, 2001 Oct;13(10):1143–7.

No authors listed. "*Lactobacillus sporogenes* monograph." *Altern Med Rev*, 2002;7:340–42.

Nobaek S, et al. "Alteration of intestinal microflora is associated with reduction in abdominal bloating and pain in patients with irritable bowel syndrome." *Am J Gastroenterology*, 2000;95(5):1231–8.

Osset J, Bartolome RM, Garcia E. "Assessment of the capacity of Lactobacillus to inhibit the growth of uropathogens and block their adhesion to vaginal epithelial cells." *J Infect Dis*, 2001;183:485–91.

Ouwehand A, Isolauri E, Salminen S. "The role of intestinal microflora for the development of the immune system in early childhood." *Eur J Nutr*, 2002 Nov;41 Suppl1:I32–7.

Pelto L, et al. "Probiotic bacteria down-regulate the milk-induced inflammatory response in milk-hypersensitive subjects but have an immunostimulatory effect in healthy subjects." *Clin Exp Allergy*, 1998; 28:1474–79.

Perdigon G. "Immune system stimulation by probiotics." *J Dairy Sci*, 1995 Jul;78(7):1597–606.

Perdigon G. "Effect of yogurt on the inhibition of an intestinal carcinoma by increasing cellular apoptosis." *Int J Immunopathol Pharmacol*, 2002 Sep–Dec; 15(3):209–16.

Perdigon G, et al. "Role of yoghurt in the prevention of colon cancer." *Eur J Clin Nutr*, 2002 Aug;56 Suppl 3:S65–8.

Pessi T, et al. "Probiotics reinforce mucosal degradation of antigens in rats: implications for therapeutic use of probiotics," *J Nutr*, 1998;128:2313–18.

Pessi T, et al. "Interleukin-10 generation in atopic children following oral Lactobacillus rhamnosus GG." *Clin Exp Allergy*, 2000 Dec;30(12):1804–8.

Probiotics Shown to Improve IBS Gut Symptoms and Anxiety

Probiotic DE111 Approved as Non-novel Food; High Soluble Form Now Available

Rachid MM, et al. "Interaction of lactic acid bacteria with the gut immune system." *Eur J Clin Nutr*, 2002 Dec;56 Suppl 4:S21–6.

Rachid MM, et al. "Effect of yogurt on the inhibition of an intestinal carcinoma by increasing cellular apoptosis." *Int J Immunopathol Pharmacol*, 2002 Sep–Dec;15(3):209–216.

Reddy BS. "Prevention of colon cancer by pre- and probiotics: evidence from laboratory studies." *Br J Nutr*, 1998 Oct;80(4):S219–23.

Roberfroid MB. "Health benefits of non-digestible oligosaccharides." *Adv Exp Med Biol*, 1997;427: 211–9.

Rosenfeldt V, et al. "Effect of probiotic Lactobacillus strains in children with atopic dermatitis." *J Allergy Clin Immunol*, 2003 Feb;111(2):389–95.

69Rosenfeldt, V., et al. "Effect of probiotic *Lactobacillus* strains on acute diarrhea in a cohort of nonhospitalized children attending day-care centers," *The Pediatric Infectious Disease Journal*, 1992;21(5): 417–419.

Salminen S, Isolauri E, Salminen E. "Clinical uses of probiotics for stabilizing the gut mucosal barrier: successful strains and future challenges." *Antonie van Leewenhoek*, 1996 Oct;70(2–4):347–58.

Sanders ME and Klaenhammer TR. "Invited review: the scientific basis of *Lactobacillus acidophilus* NCFM functionality as a probiotic." *J Dairy Sci*, 2001;84:319–31.

Schofield, Lisa. "Probiotic Popularity." *Vitamin Retailer*. August 2018: 26-30.

Sehnert, Keith W. *The Garden Within: Acidophilus-Candida Connection*. Burlingame, CA: Health World, Inc. 1989.

Shahani KM and Chandan RC. "Nutritional and healthful aspects of cultured and culture-containing dairy." *J Dairy Sci,* 1979;62(10):1685–94.

Shahani KM, Vakil JR, Kilara A. "Natural antibiotic activity of Lactobacillus acidophilus and bulgaricus." *Cultured Dairy Products Journal,* 1976;11(4):14–17.

Shalev E, et al. "Ingestion of yogurt containing lactobacillus acidophilus compared with pasteurized yogurt as prophylaxis for recurrent candidal vaginitis and bacterial vaginosis." *Arch Fam Med,* 1996;5: 593–638.

Siver R. "Lactobacillus for the control of acne." *J Med Soc New Jersey,* 1964;58(2):52–3.

Song, Danfeng; Ibrahim, Salam; Hayek, Saeed. "Recent Application of Probiotics in Food and Agricultural Science." http://dx.doi.org/10.5772/50121

Topping, Bruce. "How Can I Benefit the Most From my Bacteria." Extraordinary Health. Vol. 33: 50-53.

Trenev, Natasha. 1998. *Probiotics: Nature's Internal Healers*. New York, NY: Avery Publishing.

Tuomola EM, Ouwehand AC, Salminen SJ. "The effect of probiotic bacteria on the adhesion of pathogens to human intestinal mucus." *FEMS Immunol Med Microbiol,* 1999 Nov;26(2):137–42.

Vallianou NG, Stratigou T, Tsagarakis S. Microbiome and diabetes: Where are we now? Diabetes Res Clin Pract. 2018 Oct 17. [PubMed 30342053]

Vanderhoof JA and Young RJ. "Use of probiotics in childhood gastrointestinal disorders." *J Pediatr Gastroenterol Nutr,* 1998;27:323–32.

Vogt MN, Kerby RL, Dill-McFarland KA, Harding SJ, Merluzzi AP, Johnson SC, Carlsson Cm, Asthana S, Zetterberg H, Blennow K, Bendlin BB, Rey FE. Gut microbiome alterations in Alzheimer's disease. 2017 Oct 19 [PubMed 29051531]

Wagner RD, et al. "Colonization of congenitally immunodeficient mice with probiotic bacteria." *Infect Immun,* 1997;65:3345–3351.

OTHER BOOKS AND RESOURCES

The Book of Yogurt by Sonia Uvezian (Ecco, 1999)
A cookbook and how-to book that will convert even the most strident yogurt-hater. Uvezian explains how to make yogurt and yogurt cheese, and gives a huge number of recipes for using yogurt in everyday meals.

The Garden Within: Acidophilus—Candida Connection by Keith W. Sehnert, M.D. (Health World, Inc., 1989)
A simple but clear narration of the connection between Acidophilus and Candida for layman's understanding by a person who has written several books and articles, appeared in talk shows, TV and radio programs, and made presentations in lectures/seminars/workshops in the United States, Canada, and several other parts of the world.

Health Benefits of Probiotics by Dr. S. K. Dash, Dr. Allan N. Spreen, and Dr. Beth M. Ley (BL Publications, 2002)
An informative and educational tool for the public and students pursuing careers in food science, nutrition, bacteriology, and related areas, this book covers current research on health benefits of probiotics on digestive disorders, cholesterol, immune system, yeast infection, ulcer, cancer, acne, and much more.

Healthy Digestion the Natural Way by D. Lindsey Berkson (John Wiley & Sons, 2000)
This book gives non-drug solutions that really work for IBS, IBD, constipation, diarrhea, and other GI complaints.

Lactic Acid Bacteria: Microbiology and Functional Aspects, Second Edition by Seppo Salminen and Atte von Wright (Marcel Dekker, Inc., 1998)
This revised and expanded edition covers the taxonomy, physiology, and genetic modification of lactic acid bacteria, emphasizing their practical roles as therapeutic agents, animal probiotics, and biotechnological tools.

Natural Family Living: The Mothering Guide to Parenting by Peggy O'Mara (Pocket Books, 2000)

A good introduction to natural parenting, natural birth, and extended breastfeeding. Also check out *Mothering* magazine, of which O'Mara is editor-in-chief: www.mothering.com, or at your newsstand.

Prescription Alternatives, Third Edition by Earl Mindell, R.Ph., Ph.D., and Virginia Hopkins (McGraw-Hill, 2003)

This latest edition of my book on how to treat common problems without prescription drugs. A must for every health-conscious person's bookshelf.

Probiotics: Nature's Internal Healers by Natasha Trenev (Avery Penguin Putnam, 1998)

An excellent, in-depth resource on probiotics by the founder of Natren, a leading probiotic manufacturer.

The Yeast Connection and Women's Health by William G. Crook, M.D., with Hyla Cass, M.D., and Elizabeth B. Crook (Professional Books, Inc., 2003)

Covering vaginitis, migraines, multiple sclerosis, depression, and more, this book shows readers how they can benefit from the latest medical advances with cutting-edge information, presented in easy-to-understand language.

Better Nutrition: Natural Solutions for Healthful Living
A monthly magazine on healthcare.
900 Circle 75 Parkway, N.W., Suite 205
Atlanta, GA 30339-2941
Phone: 770-988-9991
Fax: 770-988-8399
www.betternutrition.com

The Doctors' Prescription for Healthy Living
A monthly newsletter that seeks to educate consumers on the principles of safe and healthy living.
Freedom Press
1801 Chart Trail
Topanga, CA 90290
Phone: 1-800-959-9797
Fax: 310-455-8962

www.freedompressonline.com

GreatLife Magazine
Consumer magazine with articles on vitamins, minerals, herbs, and foods. *Available for free at many health and natural food stores.*

Let's Live Magazine
Consumer magazine with emphasis on the health benefits of vitamins, minerals, and herbs.
Customer service:
1-800-676-4333
P.O. Box 74908
Los Angeles, CA 90004
Subscriptions: 12 issues per year, $19.95 in the U.S.; $31.95 outside the U.S.

Physical Magazine
Magazine oriented to body builders and other serious athletes.
Customer service:
1-800-676-4333
P.O. Box 74908
Los Angeles, CA 90004
Subscriptions: 12 issues per year, $19.95 in the U.S.; $31.95 outside the U.S.

The Nutrition Reporter™ newsletter
Monthly newsletter that summarizes recent medical research on vitamins, minerals, and herbs.
Customer service:
P.O. Box 30246
Tucson, AZ 85751-0246
e-mail: jack@thenutritionreporter.com
www.nutritionreporter.com
Subscriptions: $26 per year (12 issues) in the U.S.;
$32 U.S. or $48 CNC for Canada; $38 for other countries.

PROBIOTIC SUPPLEMENT SOURCES

UAS Laboratories
9953 Valley View Rd.
Eden Prairie, MN 55344
Phone: 1-800-422-3371, 952-935-1707
Fax: 952-935-1650
E-mail: info@uaslabs.com
Website: www.uaslabs.com

Whole Foods Market, Inc.
700 Lavaca St., Suite 500
Austin, TX 78701
Phone: 512-477-4455
Website: www.wholefoodsmarket.com
Also available at all regional locations.

Tree of Life, Inc.
Corporate Headquarters
P.O. Box 9000
St. Augustine, FL 32085-9000
405 Golfway West Drive
St. Augustine, FL 32095-8839
Telephone: 904-940-2100, 800-260-2424
E-mail: mailbox@treeoflife.com
Website: www.treeoflife.com
Also available at all regional locations.

Nature's Best
195 Engineers Rd.
Hauppauge, NY 11788
Phone: 1-800-345-BEST
Also available at all regional locations.

Select Nutrition Distributors
60 Charles Lindberg Blvd., Suite 120
Uniondale, NY 11553
Phone: 516-357-0041
Fax: 516-357-9389

Probiotics are also sold at the Vitamin Shoppe, Vitamin Cottage, and other health food stores in your neighborhood.

Note: Since not all probiotic supplements are the same, consumers should look for reputable companies selling probiotic supplements with superior strains, right potency in viable condition, and with the right formulation. The probiotic bacteria must have generally recognized as safe (GRAS) status from the FDA.

INDEX

Also Availble from Bestselling Author
Dr. Earl Mindell

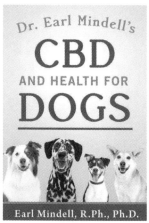

Dr. Earl Mindell's CBD and Health for Dogs
Paperback: 9781684422999
Hardcover: 9781684423002
Ebook: 9781684423019

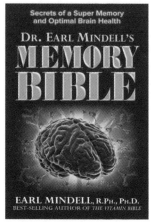

Dr. Earl Mindell's Memory Bible
Paperback: 9781591203988
Hardcover: 9781681626345
Ebook: 9781681626352

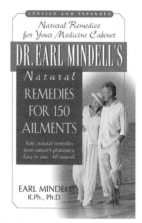

Dr. Earl Mindell's Natural Remedies for 150 Ailments
Paperback: 9781591201182
Hardcover: 9781681628998
Ebook: 9781591205845

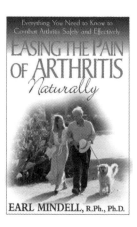

Easing the Pain of Arthritis Naturally
Paperback: 9781591201090
Hardcover: 9781681627137
Ebook: 9781591205821

Also Availble from Bestselling Author Dr. Earl Mindell

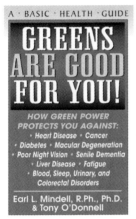

Greens Are Good for You!
Paperback: 9781591200369
Hardcover: 9781681627267
Ebook: 9781591206514

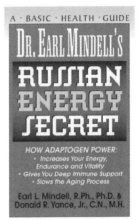

Dr. Earl Mindell's Russian Energy Secret
Paperback: 9781591200000
Hardcover: 9781681627120
Ebook: 9781591206507

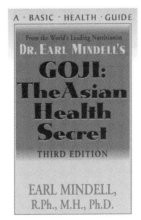

Goji: The Asian Health Secret, Third Edition
Paperback: 9781591203155
Hardcover: 9781681627243
Ebook: 9781591206231